MIX
Papier aus verantwortungsvollen Quellen
Paper from responsible sources
FSC® C105338

Dr. Divya Mittal

Imaging and Implantology

Anchor Academic
Publishing

Mittal, Divya: Imaging and Implantology, Hamburg, Anchor Academic Publishing 2015

Buch-ISBN: 978-3-95489-398-0
PDF-eBook-ISBN: 978-3-95489-898-5
Druck/Herstellung: Anchor Academic Publishing, Hamburg, 2015

Bibliografische Information der Deutschen Nationalbibliothek:
Die Deutsche Nationalbibliothek verzeichnet diese Publikation in der Deutschen Nationalbibliografie; detaillierte bibliografische Daten sind im Internet über http://dnb.d-nb.de abrufbar.

Bibliographical Information of the German National Library:
The German National Library lists this publication in the German National Bibliography. Detailed bibliographic data can be found at: http://dnb.d-nb.de

All rights reserved. This publication may not be reproduced, stored in a retrieval system or transmitted, in any form or by any means, electronic, mechanical, photocopying, recording or otherwise, without the prior permission of the publishers.

Das Werk einschließlich aller seiner Teile ist urheberrechtlich geschützt. Jede Verwertung außerhalb der Grenzen des Urheberrechtsgesetzes ist ohne Zustimmung des Verlages unzulässig und strafbar. Dies gilt insbesondere für Vervielfältigungen, Übersetzungen, Mikroverfilmungen und die Einspeicherung und Bearbeitung in elektronischen Systemen.

Die Wiedergabe von Gebrauchsnamen, Handelsnamen, Warenbezeichnungen usw. in diesem Werk berechtigt auch ohne besondere Kennzeichnung nicht zu der Annahme, dass solche Namen im Sinne der Warenzeichen- und Markenschutz-Gesetzgebung als frei zu betrachten wären und daher von jedermann benutzt werden dürften.

Die Informationen in diesem Werk wurden mit Sorgfalt erarbeitet. Dennoch können Fehler nicht vollständig ausgeschlossen werden und die Diplomica Verlag GmbH, die Autoren oder Übersetzer übernehmen keine juristische Verantwortung oder irgendeine Haftung für evtl. verbliebene fehlerhafte Angaben und deren Folgen.

Alle Rechte vorbehalten

© Anchor Academic Publishing, Imprint der Diplomica Verlag GmbH
Hermannstal 119k, 22119 Hamburg
http://www.diplomica-verlag.de, Hamburg 2015
Printed in Germany

Table of Contents

INTRODUCTION	7
OBJECTIVES OF DIAGNOSTIC IMAGING	9
IMAGING MODALITIES	11
PRE-PROSTHETIC IMAGING MODALITIES	15
PERIAPICAL RADIOGRAPHY	17
DIGITAL RADIOGRAPHY	23
OCCLUSAL RADIOGRAPHY	36
CEPHALOMETRIC RADIOGRAPHY	39
PANORAMIC RADIOGRAPHY	42
TOMOGRAPHY	54
MAGNETIC RESONANCE IMAGING	73
DIAGNOSTIC TEMPLATE	78
RECOMMENDED PRE-SURGICAL TREATMENT PLANNING	84
SURGICAL AND INTERVENTIONAL IMAGING	88
POST-PROSTHETIC IMAGING	90
RECENT ADVANCES IN DIAGNOSTIC IMAGING	98
DIGITAL SUBTRACTION RADIOGRAPHY (DSR)	99
ZONOGRAPHY	101
CONCLUSION	116
BIBLIOGRAPHY	117

INTRODUCTION

The ideal goal of modern dentistry is to restore the patient to normal contour, function, comfort, esthetics, speech, and health. What makes implant dentistry unique is the ability to achieve this ideal goal regardless of the atrophy, disease, or injury of the stomatognathic system.[33] The mere knowledge of the technique of implant treatment is not sufficient to eliminate all problems, the dentist has to be able to analyze a given clinical situation and evaluate the complexity. Acceptance of dental implantology as an integral part of conventional practice makes it necessary for the general dentist to be knowledgeable of implant imaging techniques and their clinical application.[34,38] These imaging modalities contribute information for every stage of the treatment, extending from pre-surgical diagnosis and treatment planning, through surgical placement and postoperative assessment of the implant, into the prosthetic restoration and long-term surveillance phase. So, to develop and implement a coh8esive and comprehensive treatment plan, diagnosis and imaging play a major role.[33,54]

The purpose of implant imaging is to assist the implant team in restoring the patient's occlusion and function by providing accurate and reliable diagnostic information on the patient's anatomy at the proposed implant sites. The development of precise pre-surgical imaging techniques and surgical templates allow the dentist to place these implants with relative ease & predictability.[9,34] The routine dental radiographic views and more complex imaging procedures are useful in case planning. Imaging is the integral part of preoperative implant assessment because it is one of the most accurate means by which the clinician can assess the morphologic features of the proposed fixture sites. The volume, and to a certain extent the quality of bone available for implant insertion can be anticipated from such investigations.[34,38]

Hence, diagnosis and imaging involve the participation of a number of dentists and implantologists which play an important role in developing the patient's treatment plan and objectives.[9,14]

Various imaging modalities are available ranging from standard projections routinely available in dental office to more complex radiographic techniques typically available in radiology centers. Standard projections include intraoral- periapical, occlusal radiographs and extra-oral-panoramic, lateral cephalometric radiographs. More complex imaging techniques include conventional X-ray Tomography, Computed Tomography (CT) & Cone–Beam C.T (CBCT). Often combinations of various modalities are used, as no single modality can provide all information pertinent to the radiographic evaluation of the implant patient. Awareness of benefits and limitations of the various techniques should guide the decision making process and selection of radiographic examination for the individual patient.[33,34,61]

Radiographic examination is a central part of implant treatment from the planning phase to the long-term evaluation of treatment success…….

OBJECTIVES OF DIAGNOSTIC IMAGING

DIAGNOSIS is defined as "the determination of the nature of a disease"[24]

DIAGNOSTIC IMAGING is defined as use of <u>electromagnetic radiation</u> to produce images of internal body structures for diagnosis.[24,61]

METHODOLOGY OF DIAGNOSIS[19,33,44]

1) Collection of Information
    - Medical History
    - Physical Examination
    - Laboratory Tests
    - Special Tests
2) Systemic Evaluation
3) Planning diagnostic procedures & consultations to confirm diagnostic hypothesis.
4) Complete recording and filing of collected data.

Depending on the decision of when to image and which imaging modality to be used, diagnostic imaging can be organized into three phases:[33,34,38]

1) PHASE 1: Pre-prosthetic phase
2) PHASE 2: Surgical and interventional phase
3) PHASE 3: Post-prosthetic phase

PHASE 1: Pre-prosthetic implant imaging involves all radiologic examinations to assist implant team in determining the patient's final and comprehensive treatment plan.

OBJECTIVES - To acquire necessary surgical and prosthetic information to determine the quality, quantity and angulation of the bone, the relationship of critical structures to the proposed implant site and the presence/absence of pathosis at the proposed surgical site.

PHASE 2: Surgical and interventional implant imaging focuses on assisting in the surgical and prosthetic intervention of the patient.

OBJECTIVES - To evaluate the surgery site during and immediately after surgery, optimal position and orientation of implants,

- Evaluate the healing and integration phase of implant surgery
- To ensure abutment position and prosthesis fabrication are correct.

PHASE 3: Post-prosthetic implant imaging commences just after the prosthesis placement and continues as long as the implants remain in the jaws.

OBJECTIVES - To evaluate the maintenance and function of implants including the crestal bone levels around the implant.

IMAGING MODALITIES

The decision to image the implant patient is based on the patient's clinical needs. After a decision has been made to obtain images, the imaging modality is used that yields the necessary diagnostic information related to the patient's clinical needs and results in the least radiologic risk. Many imaging modalities have been reported as useful for dental implant imaging.[21,33,34]

Various imaging modalities are: [33,49]

1) Peri-apical radiography
2) Panoramic radiography
3) Occlusal radiography
4) Cephalometric radiography
5) Tomography
6) Computed tomography
7) Magnetic resonance imaging
8) Interactive computer tomography

(I) CLASSIFICATION[54,61]

1) Two dimensional imaging modalities
2) Three dimensional imaging modalities

(II) CLASSIFICATION (ACCORDING TO PLANAR DIMENSIONS)[33,34,61]

1) Analog two-dimensional imaging modalities

2) Digital three-dimensional imaging modalities

3) Quasi three-dimensional imaging modalities

ANALOG IMAGING MODALITIES

Analog imaging modalities are two-dimensional systems that use X-ray films or intensifying screens as the image receptors. Digital images can also be produced with each analog imaging modality. The image quality of these systems is characterized by resolution or modulation transfer function, contrast H and D curve, noise / weiner spectrum, and sensitivity. The clinical performance of these imaging systems is gauged by receiver operator characteristic.[34,54]

Analog modalities[54,61]

1) Peri-apical radiography
2) Panoramic radiography
3) Occlusal radiography
4) Cephalometric radiography

DIGITAL TWO-DIMENSIONAL IMAGING

A digital two-dimensional imaging is described by an image matrix that has individual picture elements called *pixels.* A digital image is described by its width and height and pixels (i.e., 512 x 512). For larger digital images (i.e., 1.2 M x 1.2 M, where M is megapixels), the image is alternatively described as a 1.5-M image. Each picture element, or pixel, has a discrete digital value that describes the image intensity at that particular point. The value of a pixel element is described by a scale, which may be as low as 8 bits (256 values) or as high as 12 bits (4096 values) for black-and-white imaging systems, or 36 bits (65 billion values) for color imaging systems. Black and white digital images are displayed optimally on a dedicated black-and-white monitor. Generally, 8 bits or 256 levels can be displayed effectively on a monitor.[34,54,61]

DIGITAL THREE-DIMENSIONAL IMAGING

A digital three-dimensional imaging is described as an image matrix that has individual image/picture elements called **voxels**. A digital three-dimensional image is described not only by its width and height and pixels (i.e., 512 x 512) but also by its depth/thickness. An imaging volume or three-dimensional characterization of the patient is produced by contiguous images, which produce a three-dimensional structure of volume elements (i.e., CT, MRI, and ICT). Each volume element has a value that describes its intensity level. Typically, three-dimensional modalities have an intensity scale of 12 bits or 4096 values. A 3-D characterization of the patient is produced by contiguous images, which produce a 3-D structure of volume elements.[33,34]

3-D modalities

1) Computed tomography
2) Magnetic resonance imaging
3) Interactive computer tomography

QUASI THREE-DIMENSIONAL IMAGING

Quasi three-dimensional produce a number of closely spaced tomographic images and the 3-D perspective of the patient's anatomy is developed by viewing each image and mentally filling in gaps[34].

Quasi-3 D imaging

1) X-ray tomography
2) Cross sectional panoramic imaging

Commonly used radiographic procedures with time intervals for treatment planning and assessment of dental implants[61,68,74]

Stage of Treatment	Time (months)	Radiographic Procedures
Treatment planning	-1	PA, Pan, Tomo, CT, Ceph
Surgery (placement)	0	PA, Pan, Tomo, CT, Ceph for correction of problems
Healing	0-3	PA, Pan, Tomo, CT, Ceph for correction of problems
Remodelling	4-12	PA, pan
Maintenance (Without Problems)	13+	PA, Pan (follow up approximately every 3 years)
Complications	Anytime	PA, Pan, CT(as indicated)

PRE-PROSTHETIC IMAGING MODALITIES

This phase of implant imaging is intended to evaluate the current status of the patient's teeth and jaws and to develop and refine the patient's treatment plan. The global objective of this phase of treatment is to develop and implement a treatment plan for the patient that enables restoration of the patient's function and esthetics by the accurate and strategic placement of dental implants.[33,34]

The **specific objectives** of preprosthetic imaging are to:

(1) Identify disease,

(2) Determine bone quantity,

(3) Determine bone density,

(4) Identify critical structures at the proposed implant regions, and

(5) Determine the optimum position of implant placement relative to occlusal loads.

Evaluation of the patient by dentist is accomplished with a review of the patient's history, a thorough clinical examination, and a review of the patient's radiologic examinations. At this point the dentist should be able to rule out dental or bone disease and establish a tentative clinical objective that meets the patient's functional and esthetic needs. If the dentist cannot rule out dental or bone disease, further clinical or radiologic examination is necessary. The patient's functional and esthetic needs can be transformed physically into a three-dimensional diagnostic template, which enables the implant team to identify the specific sites of prospective implant surgery in the imaging examinations.[34,43,45]

In the field of oral implantology, there exist numerous radiographic imaging modalities for the pre-surgical assessment of the implant patients. In the past, intraoral radiographs and panoramic radiographs were the sole determinants of implant diagnosis and treatment planning. But with the advancement in this field, various imaging modalities are available.[33,62,68] These are further classified as:

1) Planar two-dimensional,

2) Quasi three-dimensional, and

3) Three-dimensional imaging modalities

PLANAR TWO-DIMENSIONAL MODALITIES

They are simply two-dimensional projections of the patient's anatomy. Planar imaging modalities include:

1) Periapical imaging
2) Bite-wing imaging
3) Occlusal imaging
4) Cephalometric imaging

A ***three-dimensional treatment plan*** ideally identifies at each prospective implant site the amount of bone width, the ideal position and orientation of each implant, its optimal length and diameter, the presence and amount of cortical bone on the crest, the degree of mineralization of trabecular bone, and the position or relationship of critical structures to the proposed implant sites. Thus, the modalities of choice for pre-prosthetic implant treatment planning provide high resolution and dimensionally accurate three-dimensional information about the patient at the proposed implant sites.[33]

QUASI THREE-DIMENSIONAL IMAGING MODALITIES

It includes the production of a number of closely spaced tomographic images, and the three-dimensional perspective of the patient's anatomy is developed by viewing each image and mentally filling in the gaps.[34] It includes:

1) x-ray tomography technique
2) Some cross-sectional panoramic imaging techniques.

THREE-DIMENSIONAL IMAGING MODALITIES

It enables the dentist to view a volume of the patient's anatomy. These techniques are quantitatively accurate, and three-dimensional models of the patient's anatomy can be derived from the image data and used to produce stereotactic surgical guides and prosthetic frameworks.[33,34]

It includes:

1) CT
2) MRI

PERIAPICAL RADIOGRAPHY

Periapical radiography provides a high-resolution planar image of a limited region of the jaws.[61] Two intraoral projection techniques are commonly used for periapical radiography:

1) The paralleling technique, and
2) The bisecting-angle technique

PARALLELING TECHNIQUE

The essence of **the paralleling technique** (also called the right angle or long-cone technique) is that the x-ray film is supported parallel to the long axis of the teeth and the central ray of the x-ray beam is directed at right angles to the teeth and film .This orientation of the film, teeth, and central ray minimizes geometric distortion. To reduce geometric distortion further, the x-ray source should be located relatively distant from the teeth. The use of a long source-to-object distance reduces the apparent size of the focal spot. These factors result in images with less magnification and increased definition.[28,54,61]

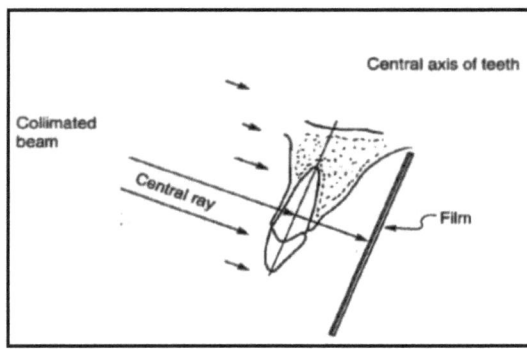

PRINCIPLE OF PARALLELING TECHNIQUE

BISECTING-ANGLE TECHNIQUE

The bisecting-angle technique is based on a simple geometric theorem, ***Cieszynski's rule*** of isometry, which states that two triangles are equal when they share one complete side and have two equal angles. Dental radiography applies the theorem as follows: Position the film as close as possible to the lingual surface of the teeth, resting in the palate or in the floor of the mouth. The plane of the film and the long axis of the teeth form an angle with its apex at the point where the film is in contact with the teeth. Construct an imaginary line that bisects this angle and direct the central ray of the beam at right angles to this bisector. This forms two triangles with two equal angles and a common side (the imaginary bisector). Consequently, when these conditions are satisfied, the images cast on the film theoretically are the same length as the projected object. To reproduce the length of each root of a multirooted tooth accurately, the central beam must be angled differently for each root. Another limitation of this technique is that the alveolar ridge often projects more coronally than its true position[28,34,61].

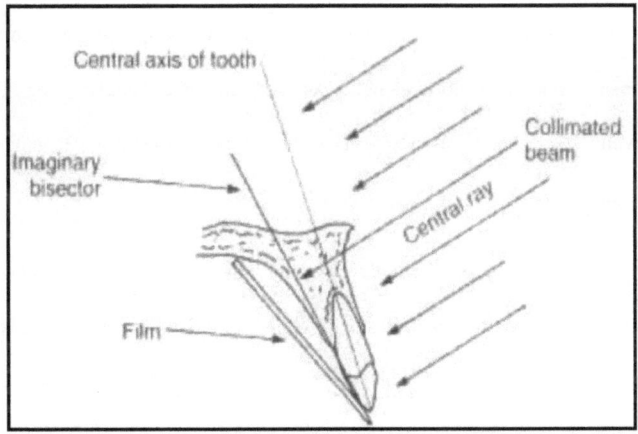

PRINCIPLE OF BISECTING-ANGLE TECHNIQUE

Most clinicians prefer the paralleling technique because it provides a less distorted view of the dentition. The long cone paralleling technique eliminates distortion and limits magnification to less than 10%. If bisecting angle technique is used then, vertical and horizontal measurements may be distorted and magnified.[32,40.61]

Image shape distortion occurs when unequal magnification of object exists. This will occur when area under consideration does not have the same focal spot to object distance. When x-ray beam is perpendicular to object, but object is not parallel to film, foreshortening will occur. If x-ray beam is oriented perpendicular to the object but not to the film, elongations will occur.[61]

No. 2 size dental film provides a 25 x 40-mm view of the jaw with each image. Periapical radiographs provide a lateral view of the jaws and no cross sectional information.

Maxillary and mandibular periapical radiographs commonly are used to evaluate the status of adjoining teeth and remaining alveolar bone in the mesial distal dimension. They may also be used for determining vertical height, architecture, and bone quality (bone density, amount of cortical bone, and amount of trabecular bone). Although readily available and relatively inexpensive, periapical radiography has geometric and anatomic limitations.[34]

The opposing landmark of available bone in implant dentistry is beyond lingual muscle attachments in the mandible or beyond the palatal vault in the maxilla. As such, the image most often must be foreshortened to visualize the opposing cortical plate. As a result, the actual available bone height may be difficult to determine by it. The bone density at the crest is also a factor to evaluate crestal bone loss with radiographic indexes.[33,38] In D4 bone, no cortical plate is present on the crest, and fine trabecular bone is primarily present. Burnout effects are common when standard kilovolt and milliampere settings are used; making crestal bone loss evaluation with digital intraoral systems is of benefit in these situations.[71] In terms of objectives of pre-prosthetic imaging, **periapical radiography** is:

(1) A useful high-yield modality for ruling out local bone or dental disease;

(2) Of limited value in determining quantity because the image is magnified, may be distorted, and does not depict the third dimension of bone width;

(3) Of limited value in determining bone density or mineralization (the lateral cortical plates prevent accurate interpretation and cannot differentiate subtle trabecular bone changes); and

(4) Of value in identifying critical structures but of little use in depicting the spatial relationship between the structures and the proposed implant site.

ADVANTAGES:[54]

1) Low radiation dose.
2) High resolution
3) Low cost
4) Minimum magnification with proper alignment and positioning.
5) Readily available.
6) High image definition.

LIMITATIONS:[54]

1) Distortion and magnification
2) Minimal site evaluation and imaging area.
3) Technique sensitive
4) Lack of cross-sectional imaging
5) Minimum reproducibility.
6) No facio-lingual dimension assessment

INDICATIONS:[54,61,71]

1) Evaluation of small edentulous space
2) Alignment and orientation during surgery
3) Recall / maintenance evaluation
4) In the preprosthetic phase, these films most often are used for single-tooth implants in regions of abundant bone width.

In implant dentistry, intraoral periapical radiographs have their application in the field of single tooth implant placement, multiple implant placement, implant placement in edentulous arch and in augmentation procedures.

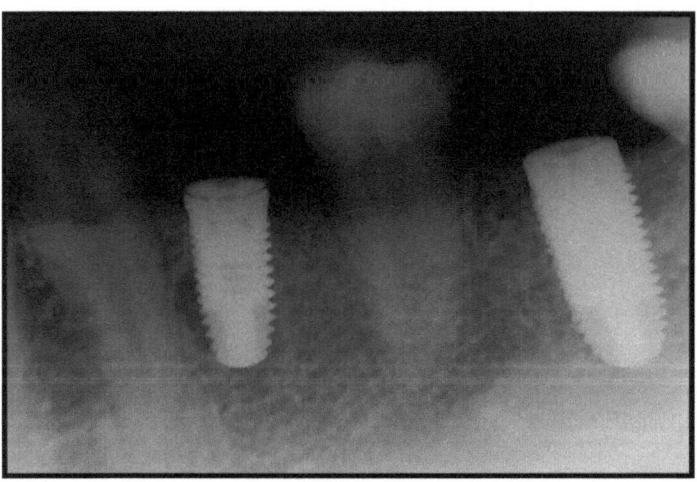

PERIAPICAL RADIOGRAPH OF IMPLANT PLACEMENT w.r.t. 44, 46

DIGITAL RADIOGRAPHY

The first digital X-ray sensors for use in dentistry were introduced in the mid-1980s by Francis Mouyen (RVG, Trophy Radiologie, Croissy Beaubourg, France [now Trophy, A Kodak Company, Rochester, N.Y.]). The first dental digital system was capable only of acquiring a radiographic image; the image could not be stored on disk but had to be printed. However simple it appeared to be, it marked the start of a new era. Shortly thereafter, another system was developed by Per Nelvig and colleagues (Sens-A-Ray, Regam Medical Systems, Sundsvall, Sweden), and within a decade many more manufacturers entered the market. Digital systems have improved considerably since then and now are a well accepted and useful technology in dental diagnosis.[48,61,66]

Digital radiographic images can be produced in different ways: flatbed scanners with a transparency adapter, slide scanners and digital cameras all can be used to convert an existing analog radiograph into a digital image. These approaches do not require a big investment, but nevertheless make it possible to bring radiographic images into the digital loop.[61,66]

Digital radiographs are of three types[48,66]:

- Direct digital radiography
- Semi-direct digital radiography
- Indirect digital radiography

In direct and semi-direct digital radiography, diagnostic imaging is produced without analog precursor.[48]

Direct digital imaging is acquired using a solid-state sensor. The solid-state sensors are based on charge-coupled device (CCD) or complementary metal oxide semiconductor (CMOS) based chips.[30,66]

Semi-direct digital radiography: Semi direct images are obtained using a phosphor plate system.[30,66]

Indirect digital radiography uses flatbed scanners with a transparency adapter, slide scanners and digital cameras all can be used to convert an existing analog radiograph into a digital image. The images produced via this technique usually are referred to as "indirect digital radiographs".[30,66]

DIRECT DIGITAL RADIOGRAPHY

It includes:

1) Charged couple device technology (CCD)
2) Complementary metal oxide semiconductor technology (CMOS)
3)

CHARGED COUPLE DEVICE TECHNOLOGY (CCD)

Most solid-state sensors in digital dental radiography are based on CCD technology. CCD refers to the design of the electronic chip that is used to capture the radiographic image. The chip converts into an electronic signal the energy of X-ray photons hitting the sensor. To increase the efficiency of this conversion, a scintillation layer is placed on top of the CCD. The scintillation layer converts X-ray photons into light photons, which then are absorbed by the CCD chip and converted into the electronic signal. This signal is sent to the computer by means of a cord between the sensor and the computer[48,61,66]

COMPLEMENTARY METAL OXIDE SEMICONDUCTOR TECHNOLOGY (CMOS)

Some solid-state sensors use CMOS technology. CMOS is not different from CCD technology in principle, but it does differ in terms of chip micro architecture. In a CMOS chip, more of the electronic components controlling the conversion of photon energy into the electronic signal are incorporated into the chip itself. This simplifies the manufacturing process and, thus, reduces the costs of production. This architecture gave CMOS an advantage over CCD for some time. However, most digital cameras on the consumer market are based on CCD technology. The quality and production costs of CCD chips have benefited from this advantage of scale, and nowadays the image quality levels of CCD- and CMOS based sensor systems are comparable.[61,65]

CCD and CMOS systems are connected to the computer by a cord. The connection can be via a wall box and the computer network. There are wireless systems on the market now, but these sensors are somewhat thicker than are systems with cords. The sensors are rigid and do not bend in the mouth of the patient and therefore could be more difficult for children to tolerate. The cord that connects the sensor to the computer may complicate the manipulations inside the patient's mouth. The image produced by a solid-state sensor is available on the computer screen within a few seconds. As a result, such systems could be efficient aids in carrying out treatment such as an endodontic procedure, in which a second image easily can be made from a slightly different angle—for example, to make the second root canal better visible—with the sensor still in the same position. This could make a solid state sensor the preferred sensor in a practice that focuses on endodontic procedures[48,66].

SEMI-DIRECT DIGITAL IMAGING

It includes:

Storage Phosphor Plate System.

STORAGE PHOSPHOR PLATE SYSTEMS

Systems using photo-stimulable phosphor (PSP)—sometimes also referred to as "storage phosphor plate"—systems use a plate covered with phosphor crystals. This phosphor layer is able to store the energy of the X-ray photons for some time. A scanner is required to "read" the image information from the plate, which it does by scanning the plate with a laser beam of near-red wavelengths. The energy is released from the phosphor layer, detected by an image intensifier and subsequently converted into digital image information. The latent image will remain in the phosphor plate before the scanning phase for minutes to hours, depending on the environment in which the plates are stored. They should not be exposed to bright light or warmth because this will release the energy before it is read by the scanner. After the plates are scanned, they are exposed to bright light that erases all remaining energy; the plates then can be used again.[26,61,66]

PSP systems are flexible to some extent, which will make it more comfortable for the patient. The plates require the extra step of the scanning procedure. The scanning time is somewhere between eight seconds for a single image and two minutes for a series of plates. Some systems take the same amount of time for the scanning of a series of up to eight plates, irrespective of the actual number of plates. The advantage of PSP is that a single scanner can be shared among several operators, similar to arrangements for a conventional film processor.[66]

EXTRA-ORAL SYSTEMS

Extra oral systems, including for panoramic and cephalometric radiograph machines, exist as well in digital versions. Both CCD-based and PSP-based systems are on the market. The advantage of CCD-based systems is the direct availability of the image. Some PSP based systems feature the ability to scan both intraoral and extra-oral plates; for others, a special scanner is required to do this. For computed tomography (CT), a PSP-system still is the only option because of the way in which the tomographic image is produced.[30,47]

COMPARISON OF FILMS v/s DIGITAL-BASED IMAGES[48,61,66]

	FILM	DIGITAL
IMAGE	ANALOG	ANALOG DIGITAL
COST	FILM,CHEMICALS	UP-FRONT
RADIATION	HIGH	50-90%LESS
VIEWING	DELAYED	IMMEDIATE
RESOLUTION	14-18Ln/mm	12-20Ln/mm
GRAY SCALE	16 SHADES	256 shades
FILM	THIN,FLEXIBLE	THIN, CORD
ENHANCEMENT	UNCHANGABLE	WIDE RANGE
STORAGE	CHART	COMPUTER

ADVANTAGES OF DIGITAL RADIOGRAPHY:[54,66]

1. Dose reduction often has been emphasized as one of the biggest advantages of digital radiography.
2. Digital radiography adheres to the ALARA principle.
3. Information recorded in the radiographic image can be made available to the observer more easily when the image is in a digital format than when it is in an analog format.
4. Computer aided image interpretation and image enhancement.
5. Standardized image archiving and image retrieval.
6. Optimum magnification
7. Excellent quality
8. Keeps aseptic setting.
9. Measurement of depth, density and neighboring structures can be done easily.

CLINICAL COMPARISON OF INTRAORAL IMAGING ALTERNATIVES[61]

IMAGING STEP	FILM	CCD/CMOS	PSP
Receptor Preparation	None	1. Place protective plastic sleeve over receptor 2. Receptor must be connected to computer and patient identifying	1. "Erase" plates 2. Package plates in protective plastic envelope

		information entered for acquisition/arching software	
Receptor Placement	1. Numerous generic film holding devices are available 2. Film may be bent to accommodate anatomy	1. Specialized receptor holder specific for manufacturer's receptor may limit options 2. Receptor inflexibility and bulk limit placement options 3. Receptor cable must be carefully routed out of patient mouth 4. Patient discomfort more likely than with film or PSP	1. Many receptor holders used for film may be adapted for PSP plates 2. Bending of receptor may irreversibly damage it
Exposure	Simple exposure	Computer must activated prior to exposure	Simple exposure
Processing	1. Dark, light – safe environment in form of darkroom or daylight loader	Image acquisition and display is almost immediate	1. Dimly light environment desirable to

29

	required 2. Processor chemistry must be prepared or replenished 3. Chemical temperature must be warmed, or processing time must be adjusted to accommodate temperature 4. Films must be removed from wrapper, lead foil must be separated for recycling		prevent loss of image information 2. Processor must be programmed with patient and detector information so that images are identified, preprocessed, and stored properly 3. Protective wrapper must be removed from plates 4. Plates must be loaded on drum systems
Display preparation	1. Films may be placed in a variety of film mounts 2. Mounts must be labeled with patient identifying information	1. Software may be configured to place image in appropriate position in digital mount when exposures are made in a predetermined	1. Images must be individually placed in mount 2. Images may need to be digitally rotated to achieve proper orientation

			sequence; otherwise, images must be individually placed in mount 2. Images may need to be digitally rotated to achieve proper orientation	
Display		1. A room with subdued lighting and a masked viewbox are optimal 2. Any light source (including the operatory window or ceiling light) will permit a quick evaluation of the image.	Same considerations apply to all digital receptor types 1. A room with subdued lighting is optimal for interpretation activities 2. A computer and display with appropriate software are necessary; viewing is restricted to the location of the computer 3. Laptop computers increase flexibility of computer placement but may reduce display quality 4. Size of the display will restrict the numbers of images that may be viewed simultaneously; more time is required to open/close or expand contact images when interpreting a series of images
Image		Quality of duplication is	1. Electric copies may be stored on a variety of

31

| duplication | always inferior to original and is sometimes non-diagnostic | media without loss of image quality 2.Output on film or paper is inferior and is often non-diagnostic unless appropriate combinations of expensive printers and papers or film are used. |

COMPARISON OF PHYSICAL PROPERTIES OF FILM, CCD, CMOS AND PSP RECEPTORS

Feature	Technical comment	Clinical comment
SPATIAL RESOLUTION	Intraoral systems: Film>CCD = CMOS>PSP Panoramic systems: Film=CCD=PSP Cephalometric systems Film>CCD=PSP	The limits of resolution for digital systems are readily appreciated when magnifying these images. With magnification a "blocky" or "pixilated" appearance is evident. Resolution of panoramic systems is limited by mechanical motion to about 1 lp/mm.
EXPOSURE LATITUDE	PSP>>CCD=CMOS≥ film	Because of the wide latitude of PSP and the automatic brightness and contract "optimization" by image acquisition software, use of more x-ray exposure than is necessary is possible.
RECEPTOR DIMENSIONS	For equivalent imaged area, Film=PSP<CCD=CMOS	The "active area" of CCD and CMOS receptors is smaller than the surface area because of other electronic components within in the plastic housing.
TIME FOR	CCD=CMOS<<PSP=film	Rapid image acquisition may be

IMAGE ACQUISITION			important for endodontic procedures or during implant placement.
IMAGE QUALITY	Subjective quality is best with film when carefully exposed and well processed.		Digital and film imaging are not significantly different when used for common diagnostic tasks.
IMAGE ADJUSTMENT/ PROCESSING	Improves appearance of digital images		Takes time; may not improve diagnostic performance
COST	Initial costs of digital systems are greater than film. Subsequent costs vary greatly depending on receptor wear and tear or abuse.		Manufacturer's estimates of life expectancy of reusable receptors are perhaps overly optimistic.
RELIABILITY	Mechanical problems affect digital PSP and film systems. Software reliability varies greatly among manufacturers. Changes in unrelated computer components and software can cause digital		Digital systems fail when problems occur with receptors during image acquisition, or with computers during image processing, archiving, and display.

		systems to malfunction.	
IMAGE STORAGE AND RETRIEVAL		Data backup is critical for digital systems	Films can be misfiled and lost or be damaged by poor storage conditions. Digital data can be lost as a result of failures in power supplies and/or storage media, as well as operator error.
TRANSMITTING IMAGES TO OTHER		Rapidly done with digital images	Facilitates communication between colleagues or with insurance companies.

OCCLUSAL RADIOGRAPHY

Occlusal radiographs are planar radiographs produced by placing the film intraorally parallel to the occlusal plane with the central x-ray beam perpendicular to the film for the mandibular image and oblique (usually 45 degrees) to the film for the maxillary image. Occlusal radiography produces high-resolution planar images of the body of the mandible or the maxilla. Maxillary occlusal radiographs are inherently oblique and so distorted they are of no quantitative use for implant dentistry, for determining the geometry or the degree of mineralization of the implant site. In addition, critical structures such as the maxillary sinus, nasal cavity, and nasal palatine canal are demonstrated, but the spatial relationship to the implant site generally is lost with this projection[54,61].

Because the mandibular occlusal radiograph is an orthogonal projection, it is a less distorted projection than the maxillary occlusal radiograph. However, the mandibular alveolus generally flares anteriorly and demonstrates a lingual inclination posteriorly, producing an oblique and distorted image of the mandibular alveolus, which is of little use in implant dentistry. In addition, the mandibular occlusal radiograph shows the widest width of bone (i.e., the symphysis) versus the width at the crest, which is where diagnostic information is needed most. The degree of mineralization of trabecular bone is not determined from this projection, and the spatial relationship between critical structures, such as the mandibular canal and the mental foramen, and the proposed implant site is lost with this projection. As a result, occlusal radiographs rarely are indicated for diagnostic preprosthetic phases in implant dentistry[61].

ADVANTAGES[54]:

1) Evaluation of pathology.

2) Provides generalized information about bone density

3) Produces high resolution imaging
4) Provides information of the inferior border of mandible
5) Laterally exposed films shows the width of the bone in midline
6) Least cost and radiation exposure.

DISADVANTAGES[54]:

1) Does not reveal true bucco-lingual width of the mandible.
2) Difficulty in positioning.
3) Degree of mineralization of bone is not determined
4) Critical structures such as maxillary sinus, nasal cavity, naso-palatine canal, mandibular canal and mental foramen can be demonstrated but the spatial relationship to the implant site is lost.
5) Mandibular alveolus generally flares anteriorly and demonstrates a lingual inclination posteriorly, producing an oblique and distorted image of the alveolus.
6) Limited reproducibility
7) Image superimposition.

INDICATIONS[9,54,61]

1) Gives information of bucco- lingual width and contour of bone
2) Helpful in assessing mandibular symphysis.
3) Individual implant site and mapping for multidirectional tomography.
4) It has its application in the field of single implant and multiple implant placements and in augmentation procedures.

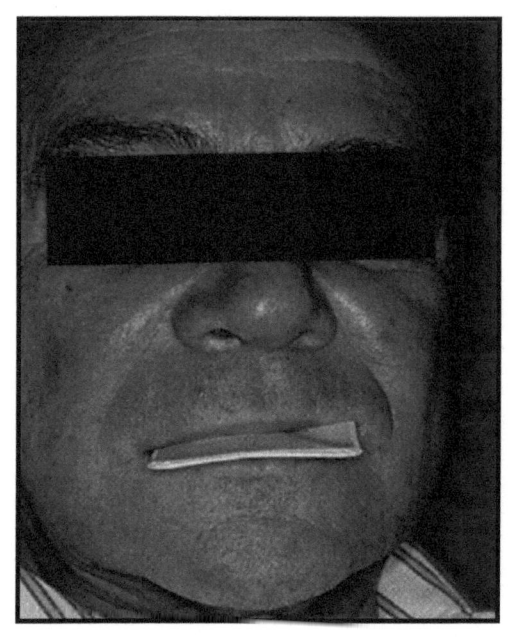

PLACEMENT OF OCCLUSAL FILM FOR RADIOGRAPH OF

MANDIBULAR SYMPHYSIS

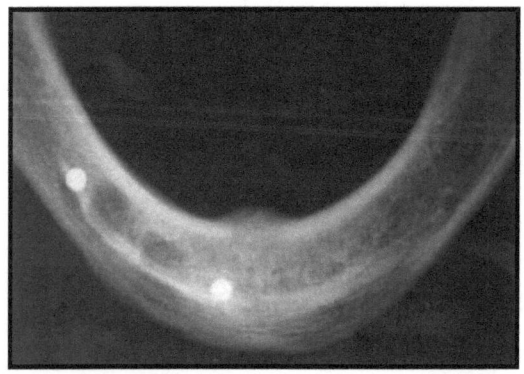

MANDIBULAR OCCLUSAL RADIOGRAPH

CEPHALOMETRIC RADIOGRAPHY

Cephalometric radiographs are oriented planar radiographs of the skull. The skull is oriented to the x-ray device and the image receptor using a cephalometer, which physically fixes the position of the skull with projections into the external auditory canal. The geometry of cephalometric imaging devices results in a 10% magnification of the image with a 60-inch focal-object and a 6-inch object-to-film distance. An image of known magnification (usually 7% to 12%) documents axial tooth inclinations and the dentoalveolar ridge relationships in the midline of the jaws. The soft tissue profile also is apparent on this film and can be used to evaluate profile alterations after prosthodontic rehabilitation.[34,54]

A lateral cephalometric radiograph is produced with the patient's midsagittal plane oriented parallel to the image receptor. This radiograph demonstrates a cross-sectional image of the alveolus of the mandible and the maxilla in the midsagittal plane. This projection can provide a cross-sectional view of only the maxillary and mandibular midline. The images of structures not in the midline are superimposed on the contralateral side, complicating the evaluation of other implant sites. With a slight rotation of the cephalometer, a cross-sectional image of the mandible or maxilla can be demonstrated in the lateral incisor or in the canine regions. Unlike panoramic or periapical images, the cross-sectional view of the alveolus demonstrates the spatial relationship between occlusion and esthetics with the length, width, angulation and geometry of the alveolus and is more accurate for bone quantity determinations. Implants often must be positioned in the anterior regions adjacent to the lingual plate.

The lateral cephalometric radiograph is useful because it demonstrates the geometry of the alveolus in the anterior region and the relationship of the lingual plate to the patient's skeletal anatomy. The width of bone in the symphysis region and the relationship between the buccal cortex and the roots of the anterior teeth also may be determined before harvesting this bone for ridge augmentation. Occasionally, lateral-oblique cephalometric radiography is used with one side of the body of the mandible positioned parallel to the film cassette. Image magnification on these views is not predictable, because the body of the mandible is not the same distance from the film as is the rotation center of the cephalostat (used to calculate object-film distance for image magnification values).[34,61]

Together with regional periapical radiographs, quantitative spatial information is available to demonstrate the geometry of the implant site and the spatial relationship between the implant site and critical structures such as the floor of the nasal cavity, the anterior recess of the maxillary sinus, and the nasal palatine canal. The lateral cephalometric view also can help evaluate a loss of vertical dimension, skeletal arch interrelationship, anterior crown/implant ratio, anterior tooth position in the prosthesis, and resultant moment of forces. As a result, cephalometric radiographs are a useful tool for the development of an implant treatment plan, especially for the completely edentulous patient. However, this technique is not useful for demonstrating bone quality and only demonstrates a cross-sectional image of the alveolus where the central rays of the x-ray device are tangent to the alveolus.[34,38,61]

ADVANTAGES[54]

1) Height/ width in the anterior region can be determined.
2) Low magnification
3) Skeletal relationship
4) Crown-implant ratio especially in anterior region
5) Tooth position in prosthesis
6) Evaluation of bone quantity in anterior region prior to symphysis grafting.

DISADVANTAGES[54]

1) Operator **technique sensitive** and if film is improperly positioned then it will lead to distorted image.
2) Image information limited to mid-line only.
3) Limited resolution and sharpness
4) Difficulty in cephalometric machine accessibility
5) Any non-midline structure is superimposed on the contralateral side.
6) Because these radiographs use intensifying screens, resolution and sharpness is compromised as compared to intraoral radiography.

INDICATIONS[54]

1) Used in combination with other techniques for anterior implants.
2) Symphysis bone graft evaluation
3) When implants have to be placed in anterior mandible.

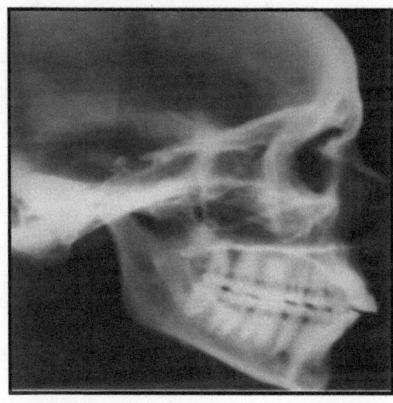

PRE-OPERATVE LATERAL CEPHALOMETRIC RADIOGRAPH

PANORAMIC RADIOGRAPHY

It is also called *pantomogram*. It is a technique for producing a single tomographic image of the facial structures that includes both the maxillary and mandibular dental arches and their supporting structures. Panoramic radiography is a curved plane tomographic radiographic technique used to depict the body of the mandible, maxilla, and the lower one half of the maxillary sinuses in a single image. This modality is probably the most used diagnostic modality in implant dentistry. However, for quantitative preprosthetic implant imaging, panoramic radiography is not the most diagnostic.[9,34]

This is a curvilinear variant of conventional tomography and is also based on the principle of the reciprocal movement of an x-ray source and an image receptor around a central point or plane, called the image layer in which the object of interest is located. Objects in front of or behind this image layer are not clearly captured because of their movement relative to the center of rotation of the receptor and x-ray source. The first to describe the principles of panoramic radiography were **Paatero** and, working independently, **Numata**.[61]

In practice, the center of rotation is located off to the side, away from the objects being imaged. During the exposure cycle, the machine automatically shifts to one or more additional rotation centers. The rate of movement of the receptor behind the slit is regulated to be the same as that of the central ray sweeping through the dental structures on the side of the patient nearest the receptor. Structures on the opposite side of the patient (near the x-ray tube) are distorted and appear out of focus because the x-ray beam sweeps through them in the direction opposite that in which the image receptor is moving. In addition, structures near the x-ray source are so magnified (and their borders so blurred) that they are not seen as discrete images on the resultant image. These structures appear only as **diffuse phantom or ghost images**. Because of both these circumstances, only structures near the receptor are usefully captured on the resultant image. Structures located more centrally in the body relative to the jaws, such as the hyoid bone and epiglottis, appear on the right, left, and sometimes central areas of final image. Most panoramic machines now use a continuously moving center of rotation rather than multiple fixed locations. This center of rotation is initially near the lingual surface of the right body of the mandible when the left temporomandibular joint (TMJ) is imaged. The rotation center moves forward along an arc that ends just lingual to the symphysis of the mandible when the midline is imaged.[34,61,67]

IMAGE LAYER

The image layer is three-dimensional curved zone (or focal trough) in which the structures lying within the layer are reasonably well defined on final panoramic image. The structures seen on a panoramic image are primarily those located within the image, layer. Object outside the image layer are blurred, magnified, or reduced in size and are sometimes distorted to the extent of not being recognizable. The shape of the image layer varies with the brand of equipment used.[61]

IMAGE RECEPTORS

Intensifying screens are routinely used in panoramic radiography because they significantly reduce the amount of radiation required for properly exposing a radiograph. Fast films combined with high speed screens are indicated for most examinations. The receptor on digital panoramic machine is either an array of charge-coupled devices (CCD) or a film-sized photo stimulable storage phosphor plate (PSP) rather than film.[61,66]

This radiographic technique produces an image of a section of the jaws of variable thickness and magnification. The image receptor traditionally has been x-ray film but may be a digital storage phosphor plate or a digital CCD receptor.

Panoramic radiography is characterized by an image of the jaws that demonstrates vertical and horizontal magnification, along with a tomographic section thickness that varies according to the anatomical position. The x-ray source exposes the jaws from a negative angulation and produces a relatively constant vertical magnification of approximately 10%. The horizontal magnification is approximately 20% and variable depending on the anatomical location, the position of the patient and the focus object distance, and the relative location of the rotation center of the x-ray system. The non uniform magnification may range from 15% to 220%.[34,61] Orthopantomography is an alternative radiologic procedure. Because of its standardized projection in the vertical plane, it is well suited for vertical measurements. Because of its complex rotational scanning mechanism, modern OPTs have been found to offer high image quality and accuracy. The inherent symmetric imaging error in the vertical plane can be corrected by the magnification factor. Structures of the jaws become magnified more as the object-film distance increases and the object x-ray source distance decreases.[61]

Structures those are located obliquely in relation to the implant receptor produce aspects of the structures that are magnified more when they are farther from the image receptor and less when they are closer to the image receptor. Uniform magnification of structures produces images with distortion that cannot be compensated for in treatment planning. The posterior maxillary regions are generally the least distorted regions of a panoramic radiograph. The tomographic section thickness of panoramic radiography or trough of focus is thick, approximately 20 mm, in the posterior regions and thin, 6 mm, in the anterior region.[54,.61]

Diagnostic templates that have 5-mm ball bearings or wires incorporated around the curvature of the dental arch and worn by the patient during the panoramic x-ray examination enable the dentist to determine the amounts of magnification in the radiograph. A technique for evaluating the panoramic radiograph for mandibular posterior implants and comparing this to the clinical evaluation during surgery was developed by identifying the mental foramen and the posterior extent of the inferior alveolar However, studies have demonstrated that the mandibular foramen cannot be identified 30% of the time on the x-ray film and when visible may not be identified correctly. The maxillary anterior edentulous region is generally oblique to the film and is often the most difficult area of a panoramic radiograph to evaluate because of the curvature of the alveolus and the inclination of the bone. The dimensions of inclined structures in panoramic radiographs are not reliable. Studies on panoramic x-ray units have demonstrated that objects in front of and behind the focal trough are blurred, magnified, reduced in size, or distorted to the extent of being unrecognizable. Information acquired from panoramic radiographs must be applied judiciously because this technique has significant limitations as a definitive pre surgical planning tool.[33,54] Angular measurements on panoramic radiographs tend to be accurate, but linear measurements are not. Image size distortion (magnification) varies significantly among films from different panoramic units and even within different areas of the same film. Vertical measurements are unreliable because of foreshortening and elongation of the anatomic structures, since the x-ray beam is not perpendicular to the long axis of the anatomic structures or to the film plane. The negative vertical angulation of the x-ray beam also may cause lingually positioned objects such as mandibular tori to be projected superiorly on the film, which may result in an overestimation of vertical bone height. Furthermore, the anatomic vertical axis varies within the film image, particularly in non midline areas. Compared with contact radiographs of dissected anatomic specimens, only 17% of panoramic measurements between the alveolar crest and superior wall of mandibular canal was found to be accurate within 1mm.[3,13,54]

Similarly, dimensional accuracy in the horizontal plane of panoramic radiographs is highly dependent on the position of the structures of interest relative to the central plane of the image layer. The horizontal dimension of images of structures located facial or lingual to the central plane but still within the image layer tends to be minified or magnified. The degree of horizontal size distortion is difficult to ascertain on panoramic radiographs because the shape of the image layer is configured to a population average and the anatomic morphology of only a few individuals conforms totally to that image layer.[58,61,67]

In 1999, **Roman G.G.et al.,** conducted a work to study the behavior of vertical and horizontal ratios in panoramic tomography in various implant regions of maxilla and mandible. Implant body was used as reference points and the enlargement was checked on adjusted radiographs vertical enlargement ratio varied between 1.21 to 1.29 and horizontal enlargement in apical end was 1.12 to 1.14 and at coronal end was 1.15 – 1.35. Results showed that enlargement variation in the horizontal ratio causes distortion of the implant body image but not in case of vertical ratio. So it was concluded that panoramic topography was suited for pre implant diagnosis, particularly in vertical dimension.

Several authors have reported that orthopantomograms (OPTs) are useful for following interforaminal implants in the edentulous mandible. Others found OPTs problematic because of the superimposition of the vertebral column on the anterior region of the maxillary and mandibular jaws and the resultant variable distortions.[58,67]

In 2001, **Dula K., et al.**, carried out a study to demonstrate that exposure risk of Periapical radiograph is 20% of that from a panoramic radiograph. Periapical and panoramic radiographs were taken of molar tooth in maxilla. Results showed that panoramic radiographs are considered the standard radiographic examination as it imparts a low dose and best radiographic image. So it was concluded that panoramic radiographic are best to assess implants especially in the maxillary region.[16]

In a study done by Zechner W et al in 2003 for the radiographic evaluation of peri-implant bone loss in anterior atrophic mandible by comparing panoramic with conventional intraoral rectangular radiographs, revealed that panoramic radiographs appeared to be comparable to intraoral small-format films in terms of the precision of evaluating peri-implant bone loss. No differences were found between the 2 imaging techniques when correlating the radiologic peri-implant bone loss with clinical parameters. Particularly in the highly atrophic interforaminal mandible, panoramic radiographic scans can be a useful alternative to intraoral periapical films for evaluating peri-implant bone loss in patients with poor imaging conditions (eg: elevation of the floor of the mouth).[67]

But **Gasser and Barth in 1987** suggested that panoramic radiographs may be superior to intraoral rectangular films in that they produce readable images of the maxillary and mandibular jaws and can be used even in patients with limited mouth opening. But they provide 2 dimensional views, which tend to be out of focus because of the superimposition of the vertebral column on the anterior region, are distorted geometrically, and magnify the structures imaged. These distortions have been reported to interfere with the evaluation of peri implant bone loss.[58,67]

ADVANTAGES[54]

1) Easy identification of opposing landmarks.

2) Initial assessment of vertical dimension of bone.

3) Convenience, ease and speed in performance in most dental offices.

4) Evaluation of gross anatomy of jaws and any related pathological findings.

5) Broad coverage of the facial bones and teeth

6) Low patient radiation dose

7) Convenience of the examination for the patient

8) Ability to be used in patients unable to open their mouths

9) Short time required in making a panoramic image, usually in the range of 3 to 4

Minutes (includes the time necessary for positioning the patient and the actual

exposure cycle)

10) Patient's ready understandability of panoramic films making them a useful visual

aid in patient education and case presentation.

DISADVANTAGES[54,61]

1) Distortions inherent in the panoramic system

2) Errors in patient positioning

3) Does not demonstrate bone quality.

4) No spatial relationship between structures

5) Misleading quantitatively because of magnification and no third dimension.

6) Panoramic radiography for linear measurements is limited because of distortion of the radiographic image.

DIGITAL PANORAMIC IMAGING (OPG)

Panoramic radiographs are the primary means of diagnosing hard-tissue disorders of the dento-maxillofacial region. These imaging methods require the use of computer-based devices that use electronic or storage phosphor receptors to record the x-ray image in a digital format. Direct digital acquisition of radiographic images provides many advantages over conventional film-based systems. Digital systems require no chemical processing system (i.e., processor unit, developing and fixer solutions, water supply, darkroom facility, and so on).[61,66]

This eliminates the inconvenience and common errors associated with film processing. Because no film has to be developed, this also makes possible the immediate viewing of the x-ray image. In addition, the environmental impact of such chemical processing has become a major concern. Because the images are in a digital format, image processing techniques can be used to enhance or analyze the image information. The cost and time of storing and retrieving digital images is considerably decreased. Finally, the higher efficiency of electronic sensors in comparison to film should make possible a substantial reduction of x-ray dose to the patient with a proportional reduction of risk.[54]

The basic principle is the replacement of the x-ray film in panoramic radiography with an electronic sensor that delivers the image information to a computer for storage in digital format. Data for successive columns of image pixels are acquired while the x-ray source and detector rotate around the head of the patient.[61]

The pixel columns are assembled to present a panoramic view of a curved plane approximating the patient's mandible. The images, which are similar to conventional panoramic radiographs, are displayed on a high-resolution video monitor and may be stored on an optical disk for future use. The solid-state linear x-ray image sensor is composed of a linear array of silicon photodiodes covered by a scintillator, which detects x-rays passing through the object being examined. The sensor has 512 elements with a 0.225-mm pitch and 0.5-mm effective width.[61,67]

A group of multiplexers successively reads out the signal from each element of the detector. An electronic preprocessor then corrects the analog offset and gain on each channel and digitizes the signal. A programmable timing circuit provides the external trigger ford detector read-out. The detector output is in the form of 8-bit digital image data, which are transferred to a high-speed programmable scanning interface integrated with a high-resolution display controller.[54,61]

An Intel 80386 33MHz personal computer serves as the host computer. The host interactively controls the data acquisition and display controller through menu-driven software. A high-resolution, 60-Hz non interlaced monitor is used for visualization of the digital image, and a thermal video printer provides hard copy output. The digital panoramic image is 512 X 1024 pixels with 256 shades of grey corresponding to a panoramic radiograph of 115.2 mm X 230.4 mm.[61]

A major advantage of this technique is its potential for reduction in radiation exposure to the patient with a very narrow linear detector array. The x-ray fan beam can be collimated to a fraction of the width used today. This could equate to a corresponding reduction in exposure to the patient.

In an era when ALARA, "as low as reasonably achievable," has been accepted as the standard for radiation exposure to patients, every effort should be made to implement new technologies that will make this standard a reality. Another advantage with this technology is its relative insensitivity to improper patient positioning. The use of a one dimensional detector array eliminates the "tomographic" effect associated with the moving film in conventional panoramic radiography. This characteristic should provide for increased image sharpness and a greater tolerance against positioning errors. A disadvantage of the technique is in radiographic shadows of overlying structures, such as the cervical spine, which are sharper than those seen in ordinary panoramic radiographs. (Another technology based on solid-state detectors has been developed.[3,13,58]

The basic principle of this system is to capture the image of a conventional radiographic screen using a signal intensifier tube (SIT) camera. The video output signal is recorded on a conventional videotape recorder. The individual frames of the video are subsequently digitized into the computer frame memory from these data, a selected image layer is reconstructed mathematically using digital tomosynthesis to create an image that represent the curved layer of panoramic X-ray. Thus the system has the capability to obtain any desired tomographic layer by repeating the reconstruction of the data from the videotape record. The system is composed of a radiographic screen, SIT-TV camera, videotape recorder, frame memory (512 X 1024 X 16 bits), MC68030-based computer with 24 megabytes of random access memory

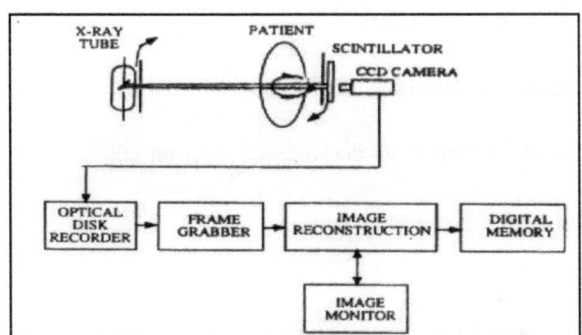

(RAM) and a high-resolution (1280 X 1024 X 8) CRT. The reconstructed image is 512 X 1024 with 256 shades of grey.[26,47,48]

Photostimulable phosphors, also known as storage phosphors, are capable of storing the energy absorbed from the x-ray beam and emitting luminescent radiation corresponding to the absorbed energy when stimulated by visible or infrared radiation. The imaging plate is exposed in the same manner as conventional screen/film systems. After the x-ray image is stored on the imaging plate, it is scanned with a helium-neon laser beam to release the stored energy in the form of light. This light is detected by a photodetector and the analog signal is converted to a digital signal that can be stored in computer memory.[26,65]

The digital image then can be displayed on a high-resolution CRT or printed to a laser printer for hard copy. The imaging plate itself can be used over and frame memory. From these data, a selected image layer is reconstructed mathematically using digital tomosynthesis to create an image that represents the curved layer of the panoramic x-ray. Thus, the system has the capability to obtain any desired tomographic layer by repeating the reconstruction of the data from the videotape recorder. The system is composed of a radiographic screen, SIT-TV camera, videotape recorder.

The basic components of the system[61] are-

1) Imaging plate - which temporarily stores the x-ray energy pattern;

2) Image reader - which converts the latent image on the imaging plate into analog and subsequently digital signals.

3) Image processor - which manipulates the image digitally and

4) Image recorder - which records the processed signal on a film.

The first panoramic x-ray machine based on "computed radiography" was developed by **Kashima and coworkers from Kanagawa Dental**. This system used a Siemens OP-5 panoramic machine and a modified photostimulable phosphor plate. Researchers at the University of Pittsburgh also have used this technique for producing digital panoramic images. The images show good spatial resolution and a wide latitude.

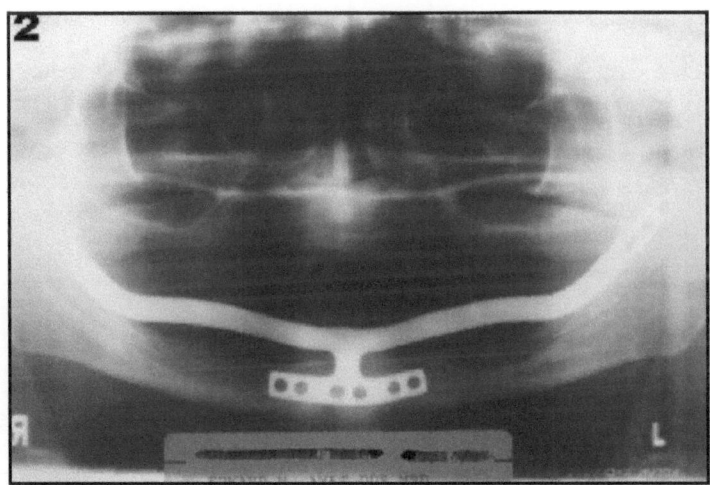

Panoramic radiograph demonstrating a mandibular subperiosteal implant.

The main advantage of this technology is that no modifications of the x-ray machine are necessary. The imaging plate is used in the same fashion as conventional film. The primary disadvantage is the high cost of the image plate and the image reading device.[58]

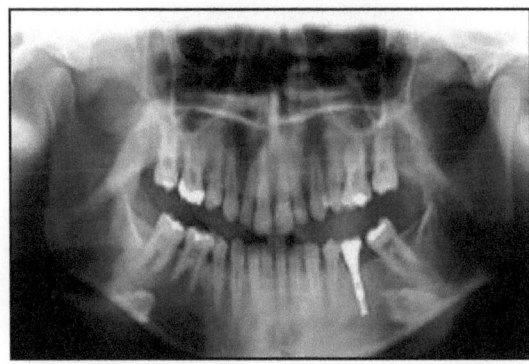

PANORAMIC RADIOGRAPH

TOMOGRAPHY

Tomography is a generic term formed from the Greek words *tomo* (slice) and *graph* (picture) that was adopted in 1962 by the International Commission on Radiological Units and Measurements to describe all forms of body section radiography. Body section radiography is a special x-ray technique that enables visualization of a *section* of the patient's anatomy by blurring regions of the patient's anatomy above and below the section of interest.[61] Many ingenious tomographic methods and devices have been developed. Tomography may be classified into many types:

1. Conventional Tomography
2. Computed Tomography
3. Three - dimensional Computed Tomography
4. Spiral Computed Tomography
5. Emission Computed Tomography

However, the basic principle of tomography is that the x-ray tube and film are connected by a rigid bar called the fulcrum bar, which pivots on a point called the fulcrum. When the system is energized, the x-ray tube moves in one direction with the film plane moving in the opposite direction and the system pivoting about the fulcrum. The fulcrum remains stationary and defines the section of interest, or the tomographic layer. Different tomographic sections are produced by adjusting the position of the fulcrum or the position of the patient relative to the fulcrum in fixed geometry system.[34,61]

Factors that affect tomographic quality are the amplitude and direction of tube travel. The greater the amplitude of tube travel, the thinner the tomographic section. Linear tomography is the simplest form of tomography in which the x-ray tube and film move in a straight line. This tomographic motion is one-dimensional and produces blurring of adjacent sections in one dimension, resulting in linear streak artifacts in the resulting image, which may obfuscate the section of interest.[54]

Complex motion, high-quality tomography is described by two-dimensional motion of the tube and film and results in uniform blurring of the regions of the patient's anatomy adjacent to the tomographic motion. Circular, spiral, and hypocycloidal are tube motions used in complex tomography.[54,61]

The diagnostic quality of the resulting tomographic image is determined by the type of tomographic motion, the section thickness, and the degree of magnification. The type of tomographic motion is probably the most important factor in tomographic quality; Hypocycloidal motion generally is accepted as the most effective blurring motion. Large-amplitude tube travel and 1-mm sections are preferred for high-contrast anatomical objects with geometry that changes in a short distance, such as the alveolus of the jaws. Magnification varies from 10% to 30%, with higher magnification generally producing higher-quality images.[1,4,34]

Dense structures such as teeth, exostoses, thick cortical plates, and dental materials/restorations are difficult to blur effectively when they are much denser than the structures depicted in the tomographic section. Dense structures may persist in the tomographic image even though they are three or four times the tomographic layer thickness distant from the tomographic section and will serve to obfuscate the structures of interest in the tomographic section.[17,22,27]

For dental implant patients, high-quality complex motion tomography demonstrates the alveolus and, taking magnification into consideration, enables quantification of the geometry of the alveolus. This technique also enables determination of the spatial relationship between the critical structures and the implant site. Ideally, tomographic sections spaced every 1 or 2mm enable evaluation of the implant site region and, with mental integration, enable appreciation of the quasi-three-dimensional appearance of the alveolus. The quantity of alveolar bone available for implant placement can be determined by compensating for magnification.[34,61]

Post imaging digitization of tomographic implant images enables use of a digital ruler to aid in the determination of alveolar bone for implant placement. Image enhancement can aid in identifying critical structures such as the inferior alveolar canal. Complex tomography is not particularly useful in determining bone quality or identifying dental and bone disease.

Conventional tomograms have a constant magnification that varies among different machines. Image magnification has been shown to be as much as 40% in some machines. Also, this technique is very operator technique sensitive with superimposition of structures outside the plane of focus causing **blurring** of the image making them difficult to read[34,61]. In addition when looking for the position of mandibular canal, vascular space and a cross- section of canal appear similar and misinterpretation is possible. Studies have shown that more than 20% tomographic images are undiagnostic.

ADVANTAGES[54]

1) Cross sectional view of site under consideration is possible.
2) Constant magnification of tomograms is there.

LIMITATIONS[54]

1) Limited availability of machines

2) High cost

   3) Multiple images are needed

   4) Technique sensitivity

   5) Blurring of image is there

   6) High radiation dose

   7) The cost of a CT scan is much higher than any other imaging system, and scanners are located mainly in large medical centers.

INDICATIONS[54]

1) Single Site Evaluation

2) Evaluation of vital structures.

3)

COMPUTED TOMOGRAPHY

The discovery and development of CT revolutionized medical imaging. CT is a digital and mathematical imaging technique that creates tomographic sections where the tomographic layer is not contaminated by blurred structures from adjacent anatomy. In addition, and probably most important, CT enables differentiation and quantification of soft and hard tissues. Thus for the first time in medical imaging, the radiologist could view hard and soft tissues on an image without performing an invasive procedure on a patient, such as the injection of contrast media.[11,17]

CT was invented by **Sir Hounsfield** and was announced to the imaging world in 1972, but it had its origins in mathematics (1917) and in astrophysics (1956). The first CT scanners appeared in medical imaging departments during the mid-1970s and were so successful that they largely replaced complex tomography by the early 1980s.[61]

CT produces axial images of a patient's anatomy. Axial images are produced perpendicular to the long axis of the body. CT is a prospectively digital imaging technique. The x-ray source is attached rigidly to a fan-beam geometry detector array, which rotates 360 degrees around the patient and collects data. The image detector is gaseous or solid state, producing electronic signals that serve as input data for a dedicated computer. The computer processes the data using back projection Fourier algorithm techniques first developed by Hounsfield to produce CT images.

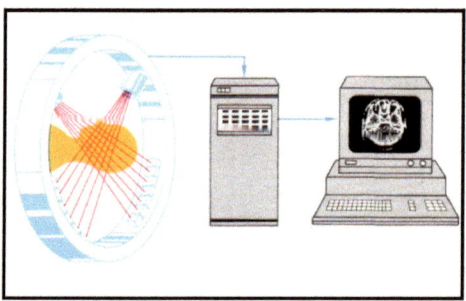

CT images are inherently three-dimensional digital images, typically 512 x 512 pixels with a thickness described by the slice spacing of the imaging technique. The individual element of the CT image is called a voxel, which has a value, referred to in Hounsfield units, that describes the density of the CT image at that point. Each voxel contains 12 bits of data and ranges from -1000 (air) to +3000 (enamel / dental materials) Hounsfield units. CT scanners are standardized at a Hounsfield value of 0 for water.[22,54,69]

TISSUE CHARACTERISATION	HOUNSFIELD UNITS
AIR	-1000
WATER	0
MUSCLE	35-70
FIBROUS TISSUE	60-90
CARTILAGE	80-130
TRABECULAR BONE	150-900
CORTICAL BONE	900-1800
DENTINE	1600-2400
ENAMEL	2500-3000

BONE QUALITY[34]:

DENSITY	HOUNSFIELD UNITS
D1	1250
D2	850-1250
D3	350-850
D4	150-350
D5	<150

The CT density scale is quantitative and meaningful in identifying and differentiating structures and tissues. CT images are inherently three dimensional. Contiguous CT images describe a three-dimensional structure of voxels. The original imaging computer can create secondary images from almost any perspective by reprojecting or reformatting the original three-dimensional voxel data. When a secondary computer is used to perform reformatting or image processing of the original CT data, the system is referred to as *a workstation.*[34,38,54]

Shahlaie. M. et al in 2003, conducted a study to evaluate variations of bone density in designated implant sites using quantitative computed tomography (QCT) and to compare the QCT measurements to subjective evaluation of bone density. Sixty-two designated implant sites in jaws of 9 human cadavers were used. Indicator rods, 2 mm in diameter, were placed in all sites. CT images representing 1-mm buccolingual slices immediately mesial and distal to the rods were selected. Bone density (in Hounsfield units) was assessed in a standardized implant area superimposed on the images and was also subjectively evaluated by 2 independent examiners using the Lekholm and Zarb classification. QCT results demonstrated that bone densities may vary markedly when different areas of a designated implant site are compared. The Lekholm and Zarb ratings for the 2 examiners showed coefficients of correlation ranging f 0.5 to 0.7 from relationships with the QCT values. Within each of the scores used for the subjective classification, however, a wide range of QCT values was observed. The results emphasize the importance of the use of radiographic methods prior to implant placement that allow topographically precise assessments of bone density in the region of interest. So it was concluded that access to QCT values should constitute a valuable supplement to subjective bone density evaluations prior to implant placement.

CT has been widely advocated for implant site assessment and is regarded as the most useful method because of its capacity to evaluate trabecular and cortical bone separately. CT may improve pretreatment diagnosis and treatment planning for implants, allowing clinicians to place the longest implant with confidence. Moreover, the fact that CT identifies various anatomical structures three-dimensionally is of great value to the diagnostician.[28,31] Although panoramic radiography measures the sum of cortical and trabecular bone whereas CT measures them separately, the high correlation of the results is attributed to the fact that measurements of cortical and trabecular bone were both included during the determination of bone density using CT. CT is proven to supply uniform images and is accepted to be reliable for performing analytic measurements.[41]

GENERATIONS OF CT[61]

1. **First generation (Rotate / Translate, pencil beam)**

    It was rotate/translate pencil beam system. Only two detectors were used, which measured transmission of X-ray through the patient for two different slices. That is two tomographic sections were taken simultaneously. It was designed specifically for evaluation of brain. In this unit head was enclosed in a water bath.

2. **Second generation (Rotate / Translate, narrow fan beam)**

    In this, a linear array of 30 detectors were incorporated. The use of 30 detectors increased the utilization of the X-ray beam by 30 times over the single detector used per slice in first generation systems. Source detector assembly intercepting a fan shaped (a narrow fan angle of 10°) beam rather than a pencil sized X-rays beam

3. **Third generation (Rotate/rotate wide fan beam)**

    The translation motion of first and second generation was a major limitation because at the end of each translation, the translational inertia developed in the X-ray tube/detector system had to be stopped; the whole system rotated and then the translation motion had to be restarted. This design could never have led to fast scanning. To overcome this limitation third generation scanners evolved. Third generation scanner uses increased number of detector (upto about 750 detector) and rotate-rotate system i.e. X-ray tube and detector array were rotated.

4. Fourth generation CT scanner rotate stationary

Fourth generation CT scanner were designed to overcome the problem of electronic drift between many detectors used in the system .Fourth generation CT scanner uses rotate only motion. Huge tube rotated but the detector assembly does not. The detector forms a ring that completely surrounds the patient. The X-ray tube rotates in a circle inside the detector ring and X-ray beam was collimated to form a fan beam.

Computed tomography provides a much more accurate to estimate of the position of the mandibular canal than does periapical and panoramic radiography and hypocycloidal tomography. For periapical radiographs, the corresponding figure was 53%, for conventional tomography 39%, and for panoramic radiography 17%. The anterior mandibular buccal depression is more readily detected on CT scans than on panoramic radiographs.[30] Computed tomographic examinations with reformatted images are the only effective means of evaluating the bone volume present below the maxillary sinuses.

Yang J. et al. in 2002, started a project to develop a light weight, simple device to evaluate alveolar process bone density using intra oral and extra oral imaging procedures. The device was constructed using barium sulphate of 5 x 32 x 12 mm^3 dimensions having eight segments of density ranging from 1.304 to 1.982g/cm^3. The device was integrated to x cp unit and placed between the jaws for computed aided tomographic imaging. The relationship between the device densities and densities of film was plotted. A linear inverse relationship was found between device segment densities and optical densities when segment densities were between 1.304 1021.882 g/cm^3 and non linear of segment densities above 1.882g/cm^3. This concluded that this device is useful for determination of material densities from 1.304 to 1.882 g/cm^3.

Several studies have been done to compare implant recipient sites by computed tomography and panoramic radiography.

In a study done by **Adkeniz, Oskan et al** in 2000, where the objective was to compare the bone height and bone density measurements of implant recipient sites by panoramic radiography and computed tomography. Thirty-seven sites of 21 patients were evaluated using both panoramic radiography and computed tomography. The data indicated that in most cases, mean bone height measurements derived from panoramic radiographs were higher than those obtained with CT images. The difference between mean bone heights obtained by two distinct radiographic methods was statistically significant ($p=0.05$). Panoramic radiography significantly underestimated the bone height compared with CT.[3]

Computed tomographic images give anatomic structures, such as cortical bone, sharper borders than do spiral tomographic images. These apparently clear borders are the result of the calculated linear attenuation for a voxel, which is the weighted average of all tissues. This effect is called partial volume averaging but may result in unreliable depictions of bone thickness and affect the reliability of measurements.[46,69]

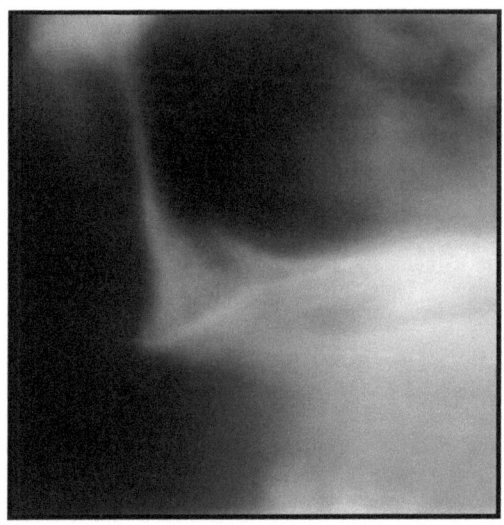

Linear tomogram of edentulous maxillary anterior region.

THREE DIMENSIONAL COMPUTED TOMOGRAPHY

The various imaging techniques applied in clinical practice are:

REFORMATTED COMPUTED TOMOGRAPHY

Patients who are edentulous or who are being considered for multiple implants and augmentation procedures may be best imaged with CT in order to investigate all possible implant sites. A lateral scout image of the selected jaw with the necessary alignment corrections for the mandible or maxilla is an essential initial step for the CT study. The jaws are aligned so that the acquired axial CT images are parallel to the occlusal plane. These axial images are thin (1~2mm) and overlapping, resulting in approximately 30 axial image slices per jaw. The image information of these sequential axial images can be manipulated to produce multiple two-dimensional images in various planes, using a computer- based process called multi planar reformatting (MPR).[61] The CT analysis results in three basic image types:

1) Axial images with a superimposed curve,

2) Reformatted cross-sectional images, and

3) Panoramic-like images.

An axial scan including the full contour of the mandible (or maxilla) at a level corresponding to the dental roots is selected as a reference for the reformatting process. The computer places a series of sequential dots on the selected scan and connects them to develop a customized arch or curve unique for each jaw. The computer program then generates a series of lines perpendicular to the curve of the individual arch. These lines are made at constant intervals (usually 1 to 2mm) and numbered sequentially on the axial image to indicate the position at which each cross-sectionals slice will be reconstructed .Cross-sectional reconstructions are made perpendicular to the curve, and panoramic (curved linear) reconstructions are made parallel with the curve. Three-dimensional representations may also be constructed in various orientations. These reformatted images provide the clinician with two-dimensional diagnostic information in all three dimensions. Typical studies provide information on the continuity of the cortical bone plates, residual bone in the mandible and maxilla, the relative location of adjoining vital structures, and the contour of soft tissues covering the osseous structures. Studies have reported that 94% of CT measurements between the alveolar crest and wall of the mandibular canal were accurate within 1 mm. Three-dimensional reformations are particularly useful in the planning of augmentation procedures such as a sinus lift and can provide an estimate of the internal density.[54,61]

The reformatted images typically are presented life size on photographic prints or radiographic film. The panoramic (curved linear) images are helpful in identifying mesial-distal relationships and non corticated mandibular canals. However, the quality of the reformatted CT study depends on the ability of the patient to remain still during image acquisition, because movement may produce geometric image distortion. Metallic restorations can cause streak image artifacts, but this can be avoided by aligning the jaws so that the acquired axial scans are parallel to the occlusal plane; thereby allowing the axial images including metallic restorations to be excluded from the study.

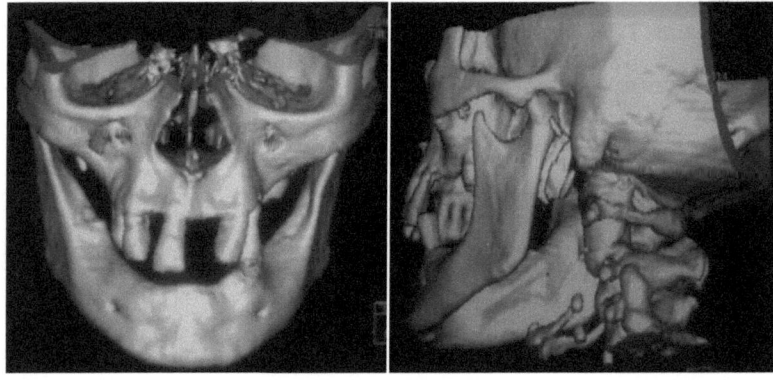

Naitoh. M. et al. in 2002 had a problem that although various panoramic X-ray machines with linear tomographic functions are now frequently applied to diagnosis related to dental implant treatment, the angles of the tomographic objective planes are automatically determined and cannot be adjusted for individual patients. To resolve this problem, a direct laser positioning (DLP) system was developed. In this investigation, the measurement accuracy of images obtained by the DLP system in comparison with those from reformatted computed tomography (CT) was assessed. A rectangular parallel piped phantom was scanned with the system and the height and width were measured on linear tomograms. Ten sites in 3 dried mandibles and 21 mandibular molar sites in 15 patients were examined both with the DLP system and the reformatted CT to compare the measured values on both images. Results showed that the difference between the actual and measured heights and widths of the phantom were within 1 mm. The difference between the values obtained by the DLP system and CT was slightly larger in the patients than those in the dried mandibles. Conclusion was that the DLP measurement accuracy was deemed sufficient for clinical use.[46]

Hence, the computed tomography, clinically helps in determining the topography of the sinus location, maximum bone depth, and the specific density of the bone at each implant site. One needs to be aware that buccal surface is always viewed on the left and lingual surface is viewed on the right side of each cross-sectional image. Thus, the cross-sectional images provide three-dimensional topography as well as bone density. The CT scan of potential implant patients is a valuable radiographic tool for diagnosis and treatment planning.[41]

DENTA-SCAN

The power and usefulness of CT for maxillofacial imaging and diagnosis were apparent as soon as high-resolution CT was introduced in the early 1980s. CT was used for imaging the temporomandibular joint, evaluating dental bone lesions, assessing maxillofacial deformities, and for preoperative and postoperative evaluation of the maxillofacial region. CT provides a unique means of post imaging analysis of proposed surgery or implant sites by reformatting the image data to create tangential and cross-sectional tomographic images of the implant site. With current generation CT scanners, reformatted images are characterized by a section thickness of 1 pixel

(0.25 mm) and an in-plane resolution of 1 pixel by the scan spacing (0.5 to 1.5 mm), producing a geometric resolution similar to that of planar imaging. The density of structures within the image is absolute and quantitative and can be used to differentiate tissues in the region and characterize bone quality[34]. CT enables the evaluation of proposed implant sites and provides diagnostic information that other imaging or combinations of imaging techniques cannot provide. The utility of CT for dental implant treatment planning was evident, but the access to these imaging techniques was limited. Access to this diagnostic information required a radiologist to communicate with the referring doctors in detail about prospective surgery and then to sit at the imaging computer or a workstation for a considerable length of time to reformat the study, interpret the resulting images, and produce hard copy images to send to the referring doctor. The advantages of this type of imaging were evident and the limitations of delivery clear, which spawned the development of a number of techniques referred to generically as Dentascan imaging[54,61].

Dentascan imaging provides programmed reformation, organization, and display of the imaging study. The radiologist or technologist simply indicates the curvature of the mandibular or maxillary arch and the computer is programmed to generate referenced cross-sectional and tangential/panoramic images of the alveolus along with three-dimensional images of the arch. The cross-sectional and panoramic images are spaced 1 mm apart and enable accurate preprosthetic treatment planning.

Limitations of Dentascan imaging include images that may not be true size and require compensation for magnification; determination of bone quality that requires use of the imaging computer or workstation; hard copy Dentascan images that only include a limited range of the diagnostic gray scale of the study; and the tilt of the patient's head during the examination, which is critical because all the cross sectional images are perpendicular to the axial imaging plane.

This technique provides a wealth of diagnostic information that is accurate, detailed, and specific. Usually a diagnostic template is necessary to take full advantage of the technique. The diagnostic template enables the dentist to incorporate the three-dimensional treatment plan of the final prosthetic result into the imaging examination; evaluate the patient's anatomy relative to the proposed implant sites, esthetics, and occlusion; and record and transfer these findings to the patient at the time of surgery.

CT enables the identification of disease, determination of bone quantity, and bone quality, identification of critical structures at the proposed regions, and determination of the position and orientation of the dental implants. Thus CT is capable of determining all five of the radiologic objectives of preprosthetic implant imaging i.e.

(1) identify disease,

(2) determine bone quantity,

(3) determine bone density,

(4) identify critical structures at the proposed implant regions, and

(5) determine the optimum position of implant placement relative to

occlusal loads

ADVANTAGES[54]

1) Negligible magnification

2) Relatively high contrast image

3) Three dimensional bone models

4) Interactive treatment planning

5) Cross referencing

LIMITATIONS[54]

1) High cost

2) Technique sensitivity

INDICATIONS[54]

1) Interactive treatment planning

2) Determination of bone density

3) Vital structure location

4) Sub-periosteal implant fabrication

5) Determination of pathology

6) Pre planning for bone augmentation

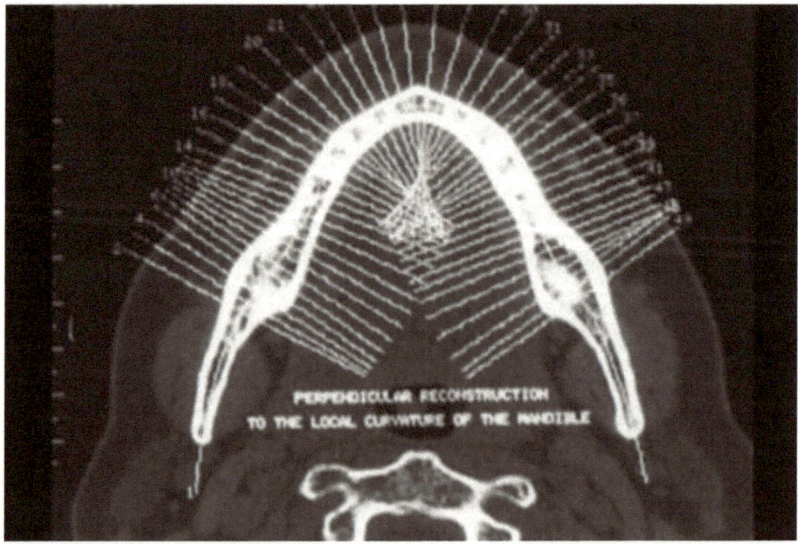

Axial CT view of the mandible showing the potential cross-sectional slices that can be reformatted by Dentascan

SPIRAL COMPUTED TOMOGRAPHY

Helical scanning uses third generation or fourth generation slip ring design. The slip ring is a circular contact with sliding brushes that allows the gantry to rotate continuously. Where examination begins, the X-ray tube rotates continuously without reversing. So while gantry is rotating, the table is moved simultaneously and data is collected continuously. This data can be reconstructed at any desired Z-axis position along the patient. By avoiding the time required to index the table acid total scan time for imaging entire patient can be much shorter. Consequently, helical scanning allows less contrast agent, since total scan time is shorter, and increase as the through but of patient through scanner. Further more in some instances entire scan can be performed within a single breath hold of the patient so that in consistent level of inhalation acquisition can avoided.[54,64]

Because patient is advancing while the gantry rotates a full 360^0 set of projection for each slice in the patient is not measured consequently to produce reconstruction of planer section of patient, the raw data from helical data sets are interposed to approximate the acquisition of planter reconstruction data.[15,64]

Kobayashi K. et al., (2004) conducted a study to evaluate the accuracy of measurement of distance on the images produced by limited cone beam computerized tomography. Five mandibles were taken and were examined by spiral computerized tomography (SCT) and limited cone beam computerized tomography (CCBCT). The distance was measured from a reference point to the alveolar ridge using a caliper and error was calculated in percentages and compared. Results show that error varied in range from 0 – 6.20% on SCT and 0 – 5.2% on LCBCT. This suggests that CCBCT is adequate for observation of bony structures and for pre operative assessment before dental implant placement.[36]

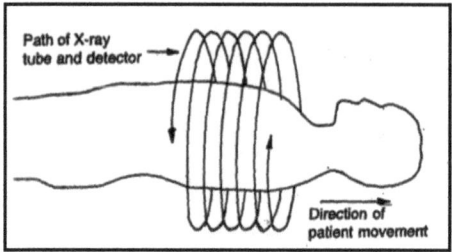

EMISSION COMPUTED TOMOGRAPHY

It provides an in vivo three-dimensional distribution of radiopharmaceuticals within the body, generated from a set of two-dimensional projection images. ECT improves image contrast and quantification. It can be divided into **single photon emission computed tomography (SPECT) and positron emission tomography** (PET).

Bambin F. et al., (2004) presented a report to assess the influence of immediate prosthetic loading on peri implant osteoblastic activity through bone scintigraphy. Implants were placed on 2 healthy women and investigated with single photon emission – computed tomography (SPECT) at 30 and 90 days after implant placement. Study was performed with planer images of ant view having immediate loading and the opposite side of mandible was control unit. Tomographic images were also taken with qualitative method. Ratios of resolution between 2 radiographic techniques were 7. Results showed that SPECT provide a direct measure of cellular activity of examined areas. So it was concluded that SPECT is an advantageous method in implant dentistry to see osteoblastic activity. And it was proved that osteoblastic activity was high in Ist6 month which declines during subsequent months.[8]

MAGNETIC RESONANCE IMAGING

MRI is a technique developed in medical imaging that is probably the most innovative and revolutionary other than CT. MRI is a technique to image the protons of the body using magnetic fields, radio frequencies, electromagnetic detectors, and computers. The technique was announced first by **Lauterbur** in 1972. Useful medical images were produced in the early 1980s, and MRI now is a cornerstone of medical imaging.[61]

Magnetic Resonance Imaging is a modern imaging modality capable of producing cross-sectional images of human body in any plane without exposing the patient to ionizing radiation. Magnetic Resonance images are produced by the interaction of the body's hydrogen nuclei, high energy magnetic fields and radio frequency pulses.[9,23]

Magnetic- Having powers of attraction (very attractive)

Alluring - Operating by means of magnetism.

Resonance -The reinforcement or prolongation of sound by reflection, as from the walls of a hollow space.

Imaging -The clinical application of an external source of energy to produce the image of internal morphology of the patients.

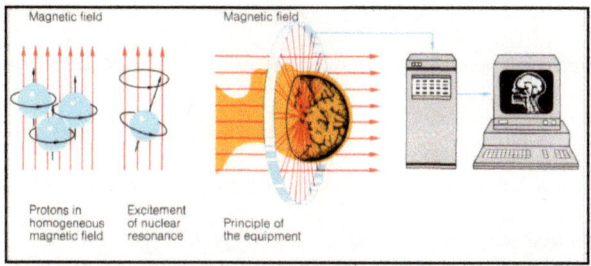

Magnetic Resonance imaging (MRI) is a non invasive method of mapping the internal structure of the body which completely avoids the use of ionizing radiation and appears to be without any hazards. It employs radio frequency (RF) pulses in the presence of carefully controlled magnetic fields in order to produce high quality cross-sectional images of the body in any given plane.[54] MRI is a three-dimensional imaging technique with an electronic image acquisition process and a resulting digital image. MRI allows complete flexibility in positioning and angulation of image sections and can produce multiple slices simultaneously. Digital magnetic resonance images are characterized by voxels with an in-plane resolution measured in pixels (512 x 512) and millimeters and a section thickness measured in millimeters (2 to 3 mm) for high-resolution imaging acquisitions[54,61]. The image sequences used to obtain magnetic resonance images can be varied to obtain fat, result of water, or balanced imaging of the patient's anatomy. The images created by MRI are result of signals generated by hydrogen protons in water or fat such that the cortical bone will appear black (radiolucent) or having no signal. Cancellous bone will generate a signal and appear white because it contains fatty marrow. Metal restorations will not produce scattering and thus will appear as black images. Thus, it is less prone to artifacts from dental restorations, prostheses and implants than CT scans. Therefore, as with CT, MRI is a quantitatively accurate technique with exact tomographic sections and no distortion. Resulting magnetic resonance images are the antithesis of CT images with cortical bone appearing dark or black and fat or water appearing bright or white. Like CT, MRI is a quantitatively accurate technique with exact tomographic sections and no distortion.[23,75]

MRI is used in implant imaging as a secondary imaging technique when primary imaging techniques such as complex tomography, CT, or ICT fail. Complex tomography fails to differentiate the inferior alveolar canal in 60% of implant cases, and CT fails to differentiate the inferior alveolar canal in about 2% of implant cases.

Failure to differentiate the inferior alveolar canal may be caused by osteoporotic trabecular bone and poorly corticated inferior alveolar canal. MRI visualizes the fat in trabecular bone and differentiates the inferior alveolar canal and neurovascular bundle from the adjacent trabecular bone[54.] Double-scout MRI protocols with volume and oriented cross-sectional imaging of the mandible produce orthogonal quantitative contiguous images of the proposed implant sites. Oriented MRI of the posterior mandible is dimensionally quantitative and enables spatial differentiation between critical structures and the proposed implant site. MRI is not useful in characterizing bone mineralization or as a high-yield technique for identifying bone or dental disease.[2,56]

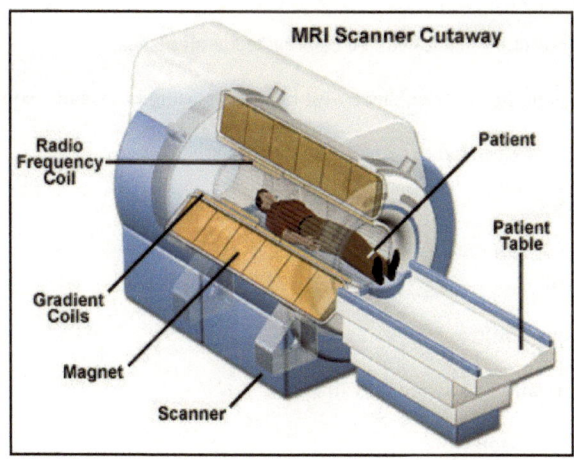

ADVANTAGES[54]

1) No radiation exposure.

2) Vital structures are seen easily (inferior alveolar canal. Maxillary sinus)

3) No biological effects due to absence of radiation exposure.

4) Higher soft tissue contrast.

5) Excellent differentiation between soft tissues is possible between normal and abnormal tissues.

6) Blood vessels clearly seen.

7) The region of the body imaged in MRI is controlled electronically; direct multi planar imaging is possible without reorienting the patient.

8) High resolution images can be constructed in all planes.

9) There is no need for enhancement of images using intravenous contrast media with their associated risks.

LIMITATIONS[54]

1) High cost

2) Technique sensitive

3) No reformatting software is available

4) Limited availability

5) Non-signal for cortical bone.

6) Potential hazard imposed by the presence of ferromagnetic metals in the vicinity of the imaging magnet.

7) Patients with cardiac pace makers, insulin pumps and ferromagnetic implants cannot be investigated by MRI.

8) Metallic objects in the oral cavity such as appliances, crowns, etc. may cause artifacts.

9) Relatively long imaging time.

INDICATIONS[54,61]

1) Evaluation of vital structures when computed tomography is not conclusive.

2) Evaluation of infection (osteomyelitis)

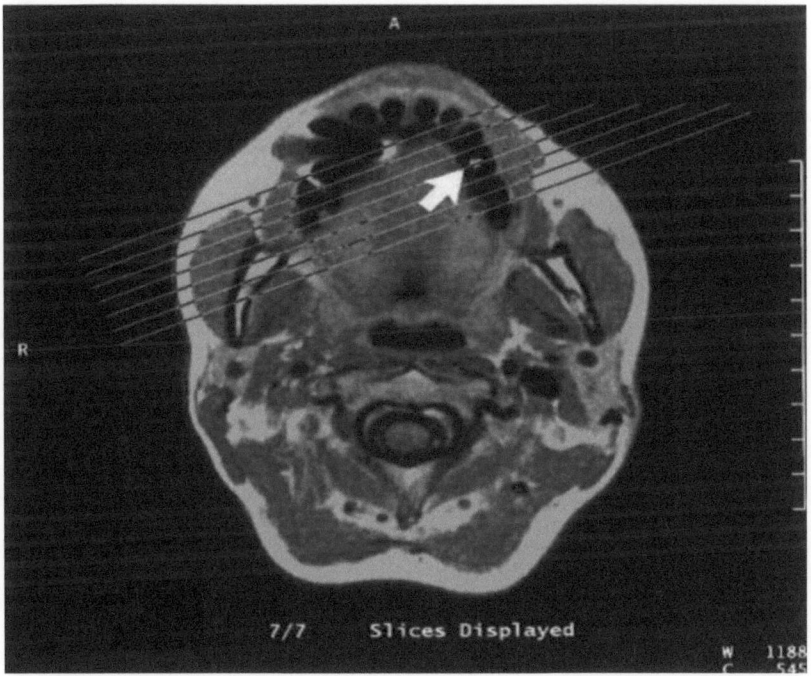

A transaxial image showing the marker indicating the potential implant site (arrow). The lines show the planned position of a set of images at right-angles to the maxilla at the site

DIAGNOSTIC TEMPLATE

The purpose of diagnostic radiographic templates is to incorporate the patient's proposed treatment plan into the radiographic examination. This requires development of tentative treatment plan before the imaging procedure. Ideally, mounted diagnostic casts, a diagnostic wax-up, agreement between the practitioners on the number and location of proposed dental implants, and prior authorization of the proposed treatment by the patient make the diagnostic template a useful tool and many times the determining factor in the final treatment plan of the patient. The preprosthetic imaging procedure enables evaluation of the proposed implant site at the ideal position and orientation identified by radiographic markers incorporated into the template.[34,54]

A stent which mimics the desired tooth setup is constructed and radiographic markers usually made of gutta percha or another radio-opaque material placed within it. Alternatively, if the patient has a suitable acrylic denture, radiographic markers may be placed within occlusal or palatal cavities cut in the acrylic teeth. The denture can also be replicated in clear acrylic to provide the radiographic stent. The radiopaque marker or rod can be placed in the position and angulation of the planned prosthetic set-up. Thus for a screw retained prosthesis the marker would indicate the access hole for the screw retaining the restoration. Alternatively the relation of the bone ridge to the proposed tooth set-up can be shown by painting the labial surface of the stent with a radiopaque varnish. The choice of radiographic marker is important in that it should be visible on the radiographic image but not interfere with the scan. When using computerized tomography (CT), metal markers should be avoided as they can produce scattering on the image .Stents are particularly useful in the edentulous patient as they also serve to stabilize the position of the jaws while the radiographs are being taken. When using CT for edentulous patients this is most desirable because of the long exposure time. The stent can also provide the radiographer with a true occlusal plane from which to orientate the axial scans. Simpler types of stent involve placing radiopaque markers e.g. ball bearings of various diameters or twisted wire shapes into a base plate and are designed to help determine mesio-distal location.[34,54]

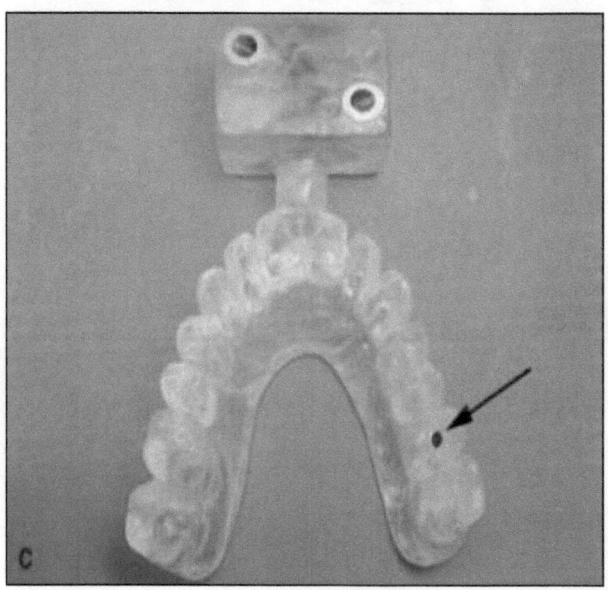

Processed stent with metal cylinders marking the implant sites

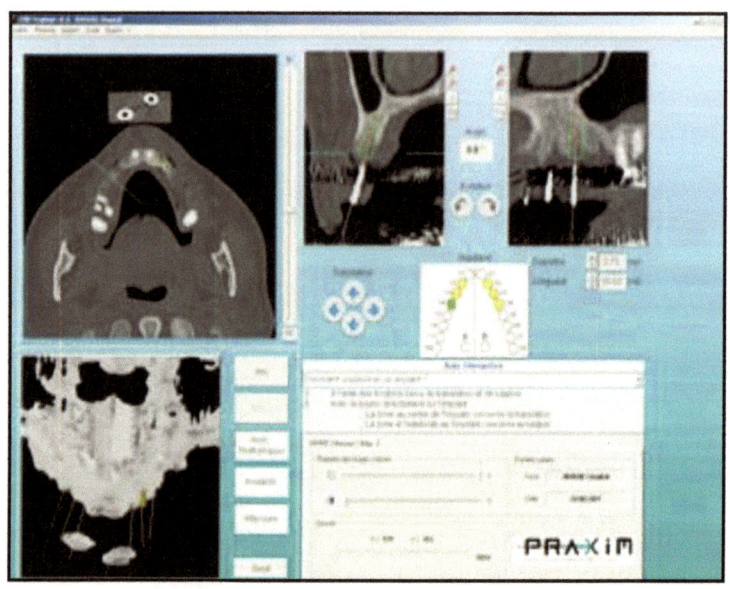

Treatment Plan Being Designed With Cad-Implant Software

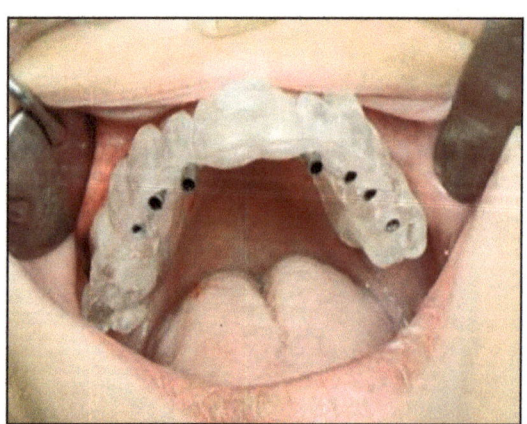

Surgical template with guiding sleeves

COMPUTED TOMOGRAPHY

The precision of CT enables use of a complex and precise diagnostic template. Although CT can identify the available bone height and width accurately for a dental implant at a proposed implant site, the exact position and orientation of the implant, which many times determine the actual length and diameter of the implant, often are dictated by the prosthesis. As such, a diagnostic template used during imaging is most beneficial. The surfaces of the proposed restorations and the exact position and orientation of each dental implant should be incorporated into the diagnostic CT template. Designs for diagnostic CT templates have evolved from a simple vacuform reproduction of the wax-up to one produced from a processed acrylic reproduction of the diagnostic wax-up and to more sophisticated types fabricated with specifically designed radiopaque denture teeth.[42,35,63]

The processed acrylic template may be modified by coating the proposed restorations with a thin film of barium sulfate and filling a hole drilled through the occlusal surface of the restoration with gutta-percha. The surfaces of the proposed restoration then become radiopaque in the CT examination, and the position and orientation of the proposed implant may be identified by the radiopaque plug of gutta-percha within the proposed restoration.[6,10]

The vacuform template has a number of variations. Another design involves coating the proposed restorations with a thin film of barium sulfate. Although the proposed restoration becomes evident in the CT examination, the ideal position and orientation of the proposed implant is not identified by this design. Another design involves filling the proposed restoration sites in the vacuform of the diagnostic wax-up with a blend of 10% barium sulfate and 90% cold-cure acrylic. This results in a radiopaque tooth appearance of the proposed restorations in the CT examination, which matches the density of enamel and dentin of natural teeth but does not identify the exact position and orientation of the proposed implant sites. The next design modifies the previous design by drilling a 2-mm hole through the occlusal surface of the proposed restoration at the ideal position and orientation of the proposed implant site with a twist drill. This procedure results in a natural tooth like appearance to the proposed restoration in the CT examination in which all the surfaces of the restoration are evident along with a 2-mm radiolucent channel through the restoration, which precisely identifies the position and orientation of the proposed implant.[33,34]

Recently radiopaque teeth specifically designed for the fabrication of diagnostic templates for fixed and removable implant-supported restorations have been introduced. The radiopaque material (barium sulfate) is an integral component of the CT scan tooth (66%to 67%). The advantages of prefabricated teeth are that they are time saving, are placed easily, provide consistently high radiopacity, have molds corresponding to prosthetic teeth used in the final restoration, and are bonded easily with the template-based material. The diagnostic template then can be modified into a surgical template.[6,7,54]

Tomography

Diagnostic templates for tomography examinations are generally less precise than those required in CT examinations. The diagnostic information available from tomography examinations is not as detailed or as precise as that available from CT examinations. The simplest tomography template is produced by obtaining a vacuform of the patient's diagnostic cast with 3-mm ball bearings placed at the proposed implant positions. A number of tomograms of the implant region are produced with the implant site identified by the one in which the ball bearing is in sharp focus. The ball bearings additionally can serve as a measure of the magnification of the imaging system, although the magnification of most tomographic imaging systems is fixed and known. Templates that incorporate metal cylinders or tubes at the proposed implant sites also enable evaluation of tomograms for the orientation along with the position of the proposed implant. The diagnostic template used in CT examinations, which is produced from a vacuform of the patient's diagnostic cast with barium coating of the proposed restoration and orthodontic wires to indicate the position and orientation of the proposed implant, also can be used for tomography and provides the most diagnostic information of the templates described.[70]

SURGICAL TEMPLATES

Diagnostic templates can be modified and used as surgical templates. If metamorphosis from diagnostic template to surgical template is the objective of the surgeon, the diagnostic template should be selected and fabricated with that in mind. Typically, bench modification of a diagnostic template to produce a surgical template does not incorporate the precision of the results of ICT or ES.

CAD-CAM STEREOTACTIC SURGICAL TEMPLATES

One can produce anatomically accurate three-dimensional models of the patient's alveolar anatomy using a number of computer-aided design / computer-aided manufacturing (CAD-CAM) and rapid prototyping procedures. CADCAM surgical stereotactic templates can be produced from CT examinations that have used ICT to develop a three dimensional treatment plan for the patient of the position and orientation of dental implant. To incorporate the three-dimensional treatment plan of implant positions and orientation into the model, the dentist also must produce the internal architecture of the patient's anatomy. The dentist then can produce a model of the patient's alveolar anatomy incorporated with the osteotomy positions and orientations.[35,70]

A stereotactic surgical template is derived from the model by aligning guide cylinders at the implant sites, which just accommodate a pilot drill, and producing a vacuform using surgical template material of the model and guide cylinders. This results in a plastic surgical template that fits and conforms to patient's bony anatomy and supports the position and orientation of the guide cylinders, which precisely reproduce the position and orientation of the proposed implants. The surgical guide is stabilized by conformation of the vacuform to the patient's bony anatomy. The stereotactic surgical template is used to establish pilot holes/osteotomies to a depth of approximately 10 mm for the position and orientation of the implants. The surgical template then is removed, and the osteotomies are completed to depth and diameter routinely.[10,59]

RECOMMENDED PRE-SURGICAL TREATMENT PLANNING

In the past, panoramic radiography was the gold standard for the dental implant treatment planning. Periapical radiographs were also used along with it. The most significant drawback to these radiographs is that they are two dimensional. For complex cases or when accurate representation and location of vital structures is needed, CT should be integrated into pre-treatment planning process[54,61].

With CT technology and interactive software, treatment planning has become very accurate modality for dental implant surgery. Because optional placement of dental implants can be challenging, special interactive software along with computer generated templates have been developed to assist implant surgeon in accurate positioning of implants. Thus, the recommended imaging for implant treatment planning is

Recommended imaging for implant treatment planning[61]

1) **DIVISION A:** Available bone with no approximate vital structures.

    Panoramic radiograph.

    Supplemental periapical radiographs, if needed.

2) **DIVISION A:** Available bone with approximate vital structures.

3) **DIVISION B:** Available bone.

4) **DIVISION C**: Available bone.

5) **DIVISION D:** Available bone(allografts, autografts , sinus grafts)

    Panoramic radiograph

    Conventional or computed tomography

    Supplemental periapical radiograph

6) **DIVISION A, B, C, D** : Available bone in which computed tomography does not clearly distinguish the exact location of mandibular canal or mental foramen.

7) Infection (osteomyelitis): MRI

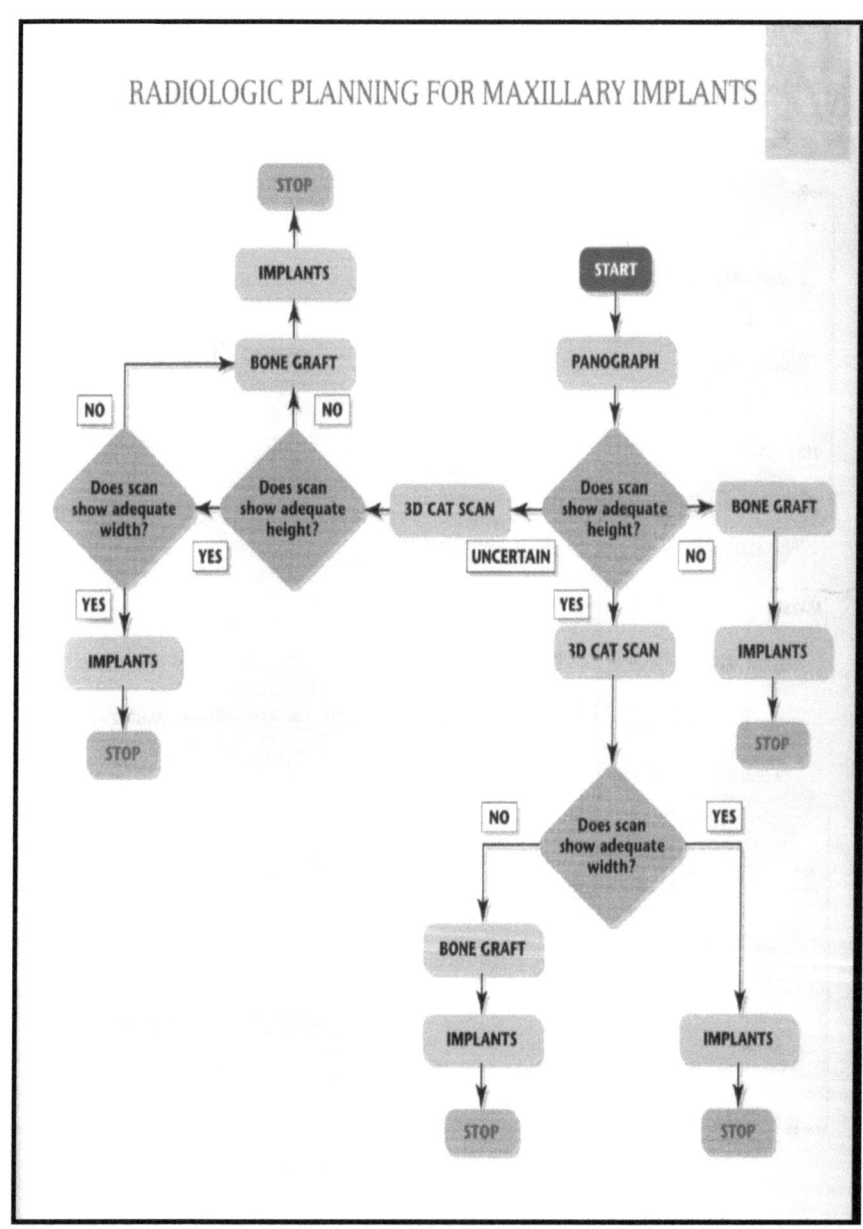

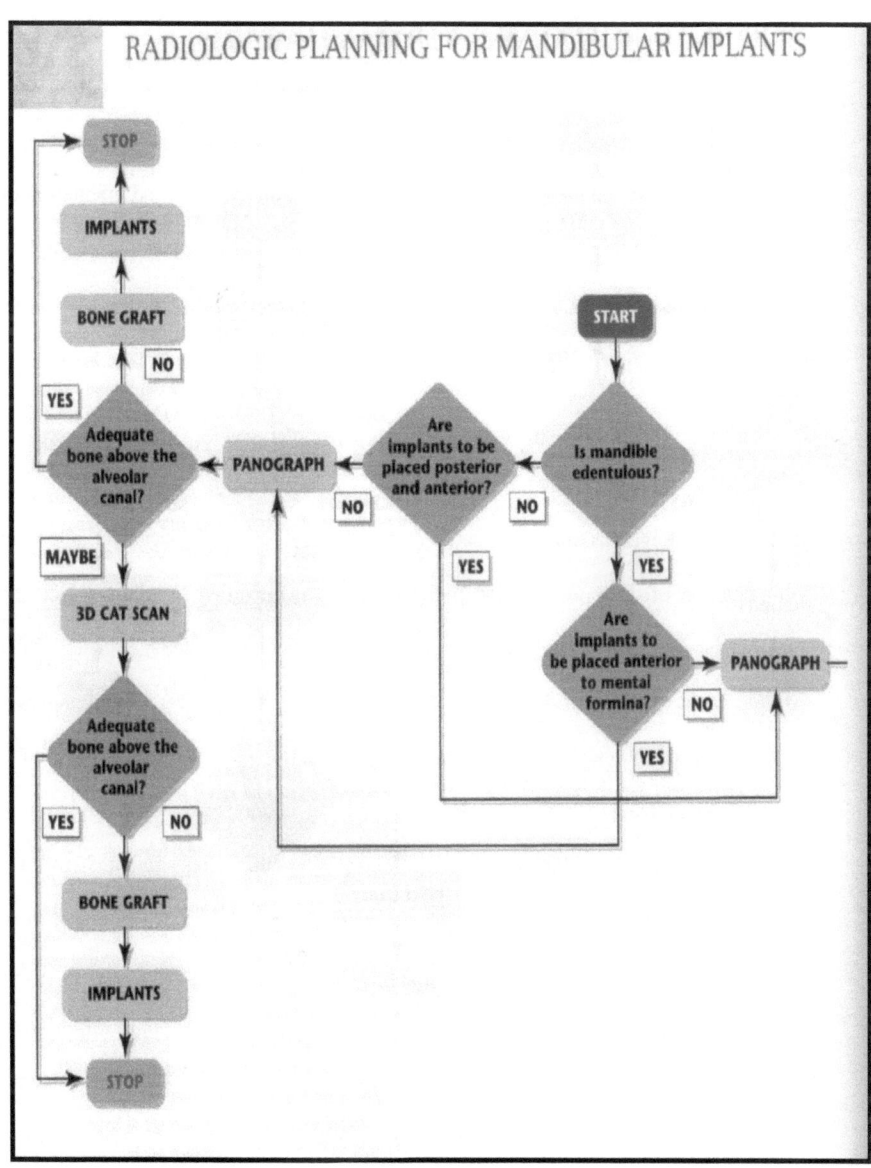

SURGICAL AND INTERVENTIONAL IMAGING

Surgical and interventional imaging involves imaging the patient during and immediately after surgery and during the placement of the prosthesis. The purpose of imaging is to evaluate the depth of implant placement, the position and orientation of implants / osteotomies, and to evaluate donor or graft sites. Because most implant surgeries are performed in the doctor's office rather than a hospital, the modalities usually are limited to[34]:

1. Periapical Radiography
2. Panoramic Radiography.

Intra-oral radiographs may be useful at the time of implant placement allowing visualization of drills or direction indicators and their relation to adjacent teeth or anatomical structures. Periapical radiographs have regained popularity because of the development of user-friendly digital radiography software that greatly facilitates peri operative implant imaging. The use of a digital sensor with a standard long cone parallel technique yields useful information during implant osteotomy preparation, especially when adjacent to existing natural teeth or other vital structures (inferior alveolar nerve, roots, maxillary antrum, preexisting features).Use of the sensor does not negate the need for a thorough preoperative radiographic assessment but provides additional information, safety, and immediate feedback at the time of surgery regarding surgical parameters such as safe zone, depth and angulation. Radiovisiography is useful as it produces an instant image at a lower radiation dose. At second stage surgery radiographs may be required to ensure full seating of abutments when direct visualization has not been possible at the time of surgery[34,54]

The patient generally can be imaged at chair side with periapical radiography to determine implant/osteotomy depth, position, and orientation. Corrections for magnification similar to those used in endodontics are necessary to quantify the depth of the osteotomy. The disadvantage of periapical radiography is that it requires a darkroom and about 5 minutes per radiograph for film processing. Digital periapical image receptors enable virtually instantaneous image acquisition, produce image quality similar to that of dental film, and enable the surgical procedure to proceed without undue delay. In addition, the digital images acquired can be viewed with considerable magnification on a video monitor in the surgery suite. Additional features of digital imaging, such as image enhancement and the use of digital measuring techniques, can help the surgeon in establishing the optimum depth and orientation of the Digital periapical and film periapical radiographs provide images of a small region of the patient's anatomy. For extensive implant procedures that may involve the entire jaw, both jaws, large donor graft sites, or sinus graft augmentation, panoramic radiography provides a more global view of the patient's anatomy[9,34].

The disadvantage of panoramic radiography is that patient generally must leave the surgical suite and stand or sit still for the panoramic procedure radiography. Panoramic radiography has less resolution than Periapical or digital periapical radiography and suffers from magnification and distortion.

Periapical or digital periapical radiographic modalities are useful to determine whether the implant components and prosthesis are seated or fitted appropriately. The antirotation devices of the implant body may prevent the abutment or impression transfer copings or any other component from seating in the correct position. This may be difficult to ascertain because the implant crest module is often at the bone crest and the tissue is several millimeters thick. A radiographic examination also is performed to determine whether the metal framework or final restoration is seated completely and whether the margins are acceptable around the implants and teeth. The important portion to image is the crestal aspect of the implant, not the apex.[34]

POST-PROSTHETIC IMAGING

The purpose of post-prosthetic implant imaging is to evaluate the status and prognosis of the dental implant. The bone adjacent to the dental implant should be evaluated regularly for the changes in mineralization or bone volume. Changes in bone mineralization in the region of bone adjacent to the dental implant may indicate successful integration, fibrous tissue interfaces, inflammation and infection, loss of crestal bone volume adjacent to the dental implant, excessive functional loading, or para-functional loading. Loss of cylindrical bone volume adjacent to the implant surface may indicate excessive axial or shear loading, bone damage during implant placement, integration failure with an epithelial bone implant interface, inflammation, or infection.[34,54]

PERIAPICAL RADIOGRAPHY

Periapical radiography produces high-resolution planar images of the dental implant and the alveolar bone adjacent to the implant. The implant bone interface is depicted at the mesial, or distal, inferior, and crestal aspects or where the central ray of the x-ray source is tangent to the implant surface. Other regions of the implant interface simply are not depicted well by this modality. Evaluating the dental implant for changes in bone mineralization or bone in alveolar bone adjacent to the implant requires evaluation of temporally acquired periapical radiographs. Interpretation of these radiographs requires scrutiny to identify changes in bone mineralization or volume that will reflect small temporal changes, which can be obscured by differences in exposure, processing, or film placement.[9,61]

BITE-WING RADIOGRAPHS

The short- and long-term evaluation of crestal bone loss around implants is evaluated best with intraoral radiographs. In these images the superior one third of the implant is the region of interest. The x-ray beam should be angled to be perpendicular to the crestal bone region of the implant or the abutment to implant connection. A vertical bite-wing radiograph is often ideal and much easier to position once the prosthesis is in place. Threaded implants make qualification of marginal bone loss easier to read. Most threaded implants have a smooth crestal region that measures 0.8 to 2 mm, depending on the manufacturer, before the threads begin, and the threads have a consistent pitch (distance between the threads). As a result, the amount of crestal bone loss can be determined by comparing the original implant insertion and initial radiograph of the prosthesis. Threaded implants also permit the doctor to evaluate the radiograph technique of the staff. The image is optimal when the implant body threads can be seen clearly on both sides.

However, if the parallel technique is poor by 20 degrees, both sides of the threaded implant will be unclear. When the right side of the implant threads (regardless of maxillary or mandibular jaw) is clear, but the left side is diffuse, the central ray was too low. The opposite occurs when the cone head is too high. When the implant threads are clear on only one side, the cone correction is approximately 10 degrees. Quality periapical or bite-wing radiographs placed parallel to the implant body with the central ray of source oriented perpendicular to the film enable sequential radiographs for crestal and peri implant bone loss. Radiographs produced in this manner should result in an undistorted image of the implant body, the implant abutment connection, and threads. Radiographs not made with this orientation produce distorted images of the implant and make interpretation and temporal comparisons difficult.[61]

TEMPORAL DIGITAL SUBTRACTION RADIOGRAPHY

Temporal digital subtraction radiography (SR) is a radiographic technique that enables two radiographs made at different points in time of the same anatomical region to be subtracted, resulting in an image of the difference between the two original radiographs. The resulting subtraction image depicts changes in the patient's anatomy, such as alveolar mineralization or volume changes, during the time between which the two radiographs were made. Subtraction radiography requires the same orientation between the x-ray source, patient, and film for each radiograph, which can be accomplished by the use of registration templates. Additionally, SR requires the radiographs to be standardized to account for changes in exposure and processing between each radiograph. Then, the radiographs can be digitized, registered, and subtracted with a resulting subtraction image that simply depicts the changes in the patient's anatomy during the time between the radiographic exposures. SR is considerably more accurate in depicting changes in bone mineralization and bone volume than simply viewing the original periapical radiograph. In addition to identifying mesial and distal changes in alveolar bone, SR also can depict buccal and lingual changes in alveolar bone. SR has been the modality of choice for depicting temporal changes of alveolar bone for clinical and research studies but had limited use in clinical practice because of the difficulty in obtaining reproducible periapical radiograph.[34,54,61]

Computed Tomography, periapical and SR techniques have limitations in determining buccal and lingual changes in alveolar bone, absolute quantification of trabecular bone, and depiction of the three-dimensional relationship between the dental implant and surrounding trabecular and cortical bone. Although CT cannot match the resolution of SR or periapical radiography, the quantitative gray-scale and three-dimensional characteristics of CT enable evaluation of the bone implant interface in all orientations. Failing implants characterized by trabecular and crestal demineralization; resorption of the bone implant interface; cortical plate fenestrations and perforation of the inferior alveolar canal, cortical plates, and nasal cavity or maxillary sinus floor can be identified with CT. CT also demonstrates the results of sinus augmentation surgery and can identify soft tissue invagination of graft sites and chronic sinus disease. Unlike conventional imaging techniques such as periapical or panoramic radiography, the resolution, spatial discrimination, and three-dimensional imaging capabilities of CT enable precise evaluation of the position of dental implants relative to critical structures such as the inferior alveolar canal, mental foramen, maxillary sinus, nasal cavity, incisive foramen, anterior loop, adjacent teeth, and buccal or lingual cortical plates.[6]

Image Modality	Applications	Cross-Sectional Information	Advantages	Disadvantages	Dose
Periapical Radiography	S,M,E,A	No	- Readily Available -High Resolution -Low Cost -Minimal Distortion	-Limited Imaging Area -No Facial Lingual Dimension -Limited Reproducibility -Image Elongation And Foreshortening	Low
Occlusal Radiography	S,M,A	No	-Readily Available -High Image Definition -Gross Facial-Lingual Dimension -Relatively Large Imaging Area -Low Cost	-No Detailed Facial-Lingual Dimension -Limited Reproducibility -Not As Applicable For Maxilla -Large Superimposition	Low
Panormic Radiography	S,M,E,A	No	-Readily Available -Large Imaging Area -Low Cost	-No Detailed Facial-Lingual Dimension -Image Distortion -Technique Errors Are Common -Inconsistent Magnification -Geometric Distortion	Low
Conventional Tomography	S,M,E,A	Yes	-Minimal Superimposition -Facial Lingual Dimension	-Less Image Definition Than Plane Films -Somewhat Limited Availability	Moderately Low, Depends On

			-Uniform Magnification -Accurate Measurements -Moderate Cost -Simulate Placement With Software	-Special Training For Interpretation -Sensitive To Technique Errors	Sites
Reformatted Computed Tomography	M,E,A	Yes	-No Superimposition -Uniform Mangnification -Accurate Measurements -Simulate Placement With Software	-Limited Availability -Sensitive To Technique Errors -Metallic Image Artifacts -Special Training For Interpretation -High Cost	High

MODALITY	RECOMMENDED TECHNIQUE	E(MSV)
INTRAORAL RADIOGRAPHY	F-speed films Rectangular collimation Paralleling technique Upper jaw: palate horizontally Lower jaw: occlusal plane horizontally	Frontal radiograph 0.002 Premolar radiograph 0.004 Molar radiograph 0.006 Full mouth survey(20 films):0.04 survey
PANORMIC IMAGING	Proper collimation Rare earth screen Proper patient positioning Meato-orbital plane horizontal Head symmetrical Lower jaw protruding Lower and upper incisors inside the image layer Neck extended Dorsum of tongue in contact with hard palate during exposure	<0.003
CEPHALOMETRIC LATERAL SKULL	Proper skull Rare earth screen Median plane of head vertical	<0.01
COMPUTED TOMOGRAPHY	KV: 120 mAs:<100 slice thickness: 1mm pitch:1-1.5suggested window:1250;level:250 Maxilla: slices parallel with hard palate from alveolar crest up to including hard palate Mandible: slices parallel with mandibular base in region of interest	

	Dose reduction by reducing number of slices, increasing pitch and/or lower mAs.	
CONVENTIONAL TOMOGRAPHY	Rare earth screen As few cuts as possible Proper positioning: The tomographic plane parallel to hard palate(maxilla) and the mandibular canal (mandible) and at the same time perpendicular to the tangent of alveolar process in the region of interest.	Maxilla<0.02 cut Mandible<0.03 cut

RECENT ADVANCES IN DIAGNOSTIC IMAGING

The increase in the popularity of and the demand for the use of dental implants to replace teeth has encouraged advancement in clinical technology and materials to improve patients' acceptance and clinical outcomes. Recent advances play a major role in the success of implant dentistry. The various recent advances in the field of diagnostic imaging in implantology are:

1) DIGITAL SUBSTRACTION RADIOGRPHY
2) ZONOGRAPHY
3) CONE BEAM VOLUMETRIC TOMOGRAPHY
4) INTERACTIVE COMPUTED TOMOGRAPHY
5) SIMPLANTS
6) SCANORA
7) CONE BEAM COMPUTED TOMOGRAPHY

DIGITAL SUBTRACTION RADIOGRAPHY (DSR)

More advanced image processing is available to dental practitioners as well. Subtraction radiography originally was described by Ziedses des Plantes in the 1930s. Webber and colleagues and Gröndahl and colleagues introduced digital subtraction into dental radiography. Subtraction radiography is able to show small differences between radiographs taken a specified time apart. This is a specialized digital technique in which two digital radiographic images of the same region are made by standardized method with an interval, one before any particular treatment and other after treatment, & then the two images are superimposed. Hence, two standard radiographs are produced with identical exposure geometry. The first one is considered as a 'reference image' and the second one is the image to be compared. These are digitized and the second image is superimposed over the test image Subtraction of the pixel values of two images with the same projection geometry shows the differences and suppresses the structures of both images that are similar, which also is called "anatomical noise". The two images used for subtraction radiography must have identical projection geometry. Otherwise, the subtraction image shows the difference of the projection geometry instead of the difference between the first and the second exposure. Several reports have been published showing how to obtain identical images, based mainly on the use of film holders connected to individual bite-blocks. Recently, however, special software is used to subtract the regions that are unchanged and thereby highlighting those regions where there is a difference. If there is a change in the radiographic attenuation between the baseline and the follow–up examination, the change shows up as brighter area when the change represents gain and as a darker area when the change represents loss.30,48,61

MECHANISM

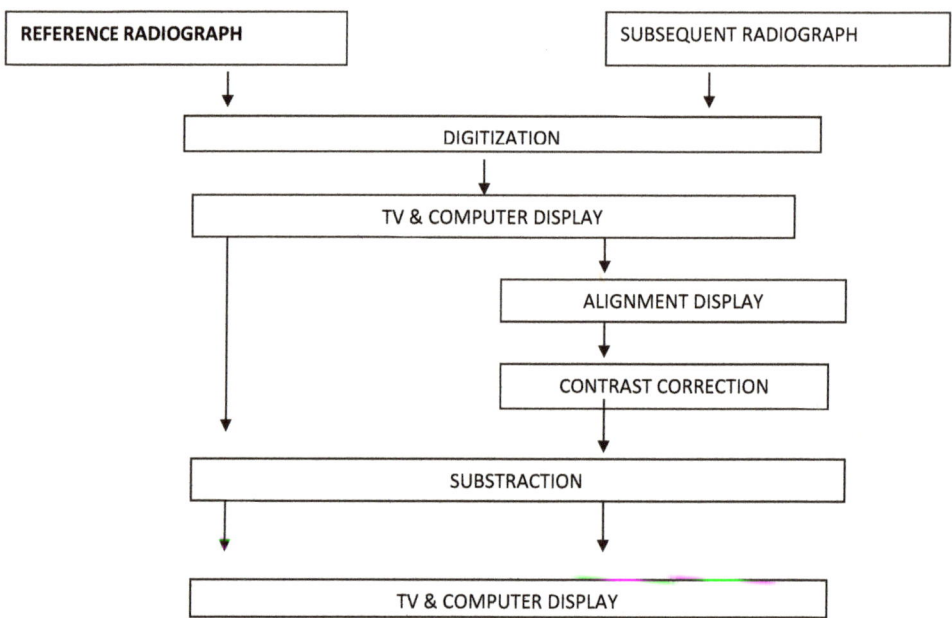

ADVANTAGES[66]

1) It cancels out the complex anatomic background against which these changes occur. This helps to increase the conspicuousness of the change.
2) With conventional radiography, it is impossible to detect a 0.85 mm changes in cortical bone thickness but digital subtraction radiography is so sensitive that it can detect 0.12 mm change.

Digital subtraction radiography can be used:

1) In periodontal and carious lesions.
2) For evaluation of small changes in mandibular condyle position and integrity of the articular surface.
3) For assessment of osseous remodeling around granular hydroxyapatite implants.

4) It has been demonstrated that the proximal carious lesions are clearly visible with DSR technique and also for detecting progress of remineralized and demineralized patterns of caries.

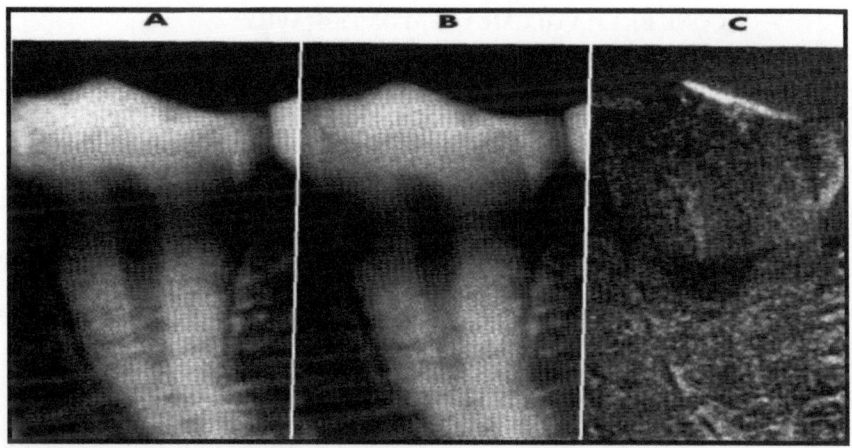

Digital subtraction radiographs. Subtraction radiography requires two images (A and B), which are exposed with the same geometry. In this instance the loss of alveolar bone in B is too subtle to be seen. However, the subtracted image (C) displays the differences between A and B; the bone loss is seen as a dark structure superimposed over the pulp.

ZONOGRAPHY

Recently a modification of the panoramic x-ray machine has been developed that has the capability of making a cross-sectional image of the jaws. These devices use limited **angle linear tomography (zonography)** and a means for positioning the patient. The tomographic layer is approximately 5 mm. This technique enables the appreciation of spatial relationship between the critical structures and the implant site and quantification of the geometry of the implant site. The tomographic layers are thick and have adjacent structures that are blurred and superimposed on the image, limiting the usefulness of this technique for individual sites, especially in the anterior regions where the geometry of the alveolus changes rapidly. This technique is not useful for determining the differences in most bone densities or identifying disease at the implant site.[34,61]

CONE BEAM VOLUMETRIC TOMOGRAPHY

A new type of advanced tomographic technique specifically developed for dental applications is *cone beam volumetric tomography* (CBVT). Because conventional computed tomography is associated with high dose of radiation, the advent of CBVT has overcome this major drawback of conventional CT. Recently with the approval of cone beam technology by US Food and Drug Administration there are more choices.[65]

INTERACTIVE COMPUTED TOMOGRAPHY

Interactive CT addresses many of the limitations of CT. ICT is a technique that was developed to bridge the gap in information transfer between the radiologist and the practitioner. Interactive computer software programs now allow reformatted CT data to be analyzed on a personal computer when developing a treatment plan. This technique enables the radiologist to transfer the imaging study to the practitioner as a computer file and enables the practitioner to view and interact with the imaging study on a personal computer. The dentist's computer becomes a diagnostic radiologic workstation, with tools to measure the length and the width of the alveolus, measure bone quality, and change the window and level of the gray scale of the study to enhance the perception of critical structures.

Axial, cross-sectional, and panoramic images are displayed and referenced so that the dentist can appreciate the same position or region within the patient's anatomy in each of the images. Regions of the patient's anatomy can be selected for display normally, with magnification, or with a number of gray-scale depictions facilitating the appreciation of anatomy, structures, or disease.[55]

An important feature of ICT is that the dentist and radiologist can perform electronic surgery by selecting and placing arbitrary-size cylinders that simulate root-form implants in the images: With an appropriately designed diagnostic template, ES can be performed to develop the Electronic implants can be placed at arbitrary positions and orientations with respect to each other, the alveolus, critical structures, and the prospective occlusion and esthetics. ES and ICT enable the development of a three-dimensional treatment plan that is integrated with the patient's anatomy and can be visualized before surgery by members of the implant team and the patient for approval or modification.[54]

ICT enables the determination of bone quality adjacent to the prospective implant sites With the number and size of implants accurately determined, along with the density of bone at the proposed implant sites, the dentist can determine the characteristics of the implants accurately before surgery.

The first step in the ICT process is impression for the study casts. With the use of these casts, diagnostic wax-up is completed according to ideal position of the missing tooth in question with emphasis on the final prosthesis. From the diagnostic wax-up, radiographic template is fabricated that patient will wear during the scan. The diagnostic template will allow the transfer of ideal positioning of the teeth that will be transformed into radiographic examination.

ICT is currently the most accurate imaging technique for implant imaging and surgery but has some limitations. ES enables placement of electronic implants in the imaging study but the refinement and exact relative orientation of the implant positions are difficult and cumbersome. For instance, three consecutive implants may require parallelism and interproximal spacing of 2.7 mm. The dentist may struggle in achieving the exact relative spacing and orientation with ES and ICT. Parallelism is difficult to appreciate in ICT using orthogonal rather than three-dimensional images. In this case, implant orientation must be deferred to the orientation developed in the diagnostic template rather than that from the images. Once the treatment plan has been developed using ICT and ES and has been approved by the implant team and the patient, executing the plan may be difficult. The precision and accuracy of the treatment plan achieved using ICT and ES for the implant position, size, orientation, relative spacing, spatial relationship to the critical structures and proposed esthetics, and occlusion become a major challenge at the time of surgery. The treatment plan may require implant positions to an accuracy of a few tenths of a millimeter and orientation to a couple of degrees. Transfer of the plan to the patient at the time of surgery can be accomplished by simple visualization and comprehension by a skilled and experienced surgeon, using positions and orientations obtained from ICT and ES to convert the diagnostic template into a surgical template or the production of a computer generated, three-dimensional stereotactic surgical template from the digital ICT and ES data.[34,54]

SIMPLANTS

SimPlant offers a complete solution in the field of dental implantology. It combines a variety of products that assures highly satisfying aesthetic results, allows minimally invasive surgery and immediate loading and enhances the predictability of the overall working procedure. A recently developed interactive 3-dimensional CT software program (SimPlant; Materialse, Leuven, Belgium) has made it possible to visualize the anatomical structures in a 3-dimensional mode on computer monitors for interactive implant placement. SimPlant uses raw data (DICOM files) from the CT scan to display reformatted CT images for the inspection of the bony anatomy of the alveolar ridges. Bone height and width can be easily measured from point to point. The planned implant length and diameter can therefore be determined. The angulation of the planned implant can be adjusted for optimal orientation with respect to the natural teeth and bony anatomy. The esthetic and biomechanical considerations (implant alignment) are made easier with 3-dimensional images. These interactive, reformatted cross-sectional images, used together with 3-dimensional reconstruction planning, give a better prognostic value than conventional reformatted cross-sectional CT planning for implant lengths. The CT scan data obtained from the SimPlant software can be used to produce sterolithographic models for 3-dimensional visualization for planning complex maxillofacial surgery.[10,59] There are two techniques available for making sterolithographic models. The first technique applies laser technology in which a sterolithographic model is built up, layer by layer, with resin solution. A resin layer is solidified when its surface is struck with the laser. Another technique uses a computer-aided milling machine. Surgical guides, and provisional and permanent restorations for implants, can all be fabricated using sterolithographic models.[20,70]

SimPlant comprises the following products: SimPlant software, SurgiGuide drill guides, the SAFE system, and the Immediate Smile concept. SimPlant is precise preoperative planning software to accurately plan the placement of dental implants. Because SimPlant integrates data from a CT scan, it provides precise information on the anatomy of the patient. The software allows treatment planning for the ideal position of the implants in both 2D and 3D, while taking into account clinical and aesthetical considerations. The precise treatment plan made with SimPlant can be transferred to surgery with SurgiGuide drill guides. SurgiGuide drill guides are custom-made, patient specific surgical drill guides made from the SimPlant treatment plan. SurgiGuide drill guides guide the drill during surgery to the exact implant location and the exact angulation as planned. SurgiGuide drill guides are available as bone-supported, tooth-supported or mucosa-supported to accommodate all surgical preferences.[42,59] The SAFE System (Secure, Accurate, Flexible, Ergonomic) takes SurgiGuide drill guides to the next level. SAFE is the latest development in SimPlant, enhancing the predictability and accuracy of implant dentistry. The system combines drilling guidance with depth control and implant insertion. This highly accurate system opens the door to immediate loading cases. Materialize Dental's immediate loading concept, called Immediate Smile enables the implant clinician to have the prosthesis pre-manufactured for surgery and makes implant surgery and restoration possible in one appointment.

PRINCIPLE

Axial CT scans are post processes using software program; the reformatted Dental scan type images can be manipulated by SimPlant. The formatted CT study can be transmitted to the implant clinician in non compressed form in floppy disk or by email. After downloading the data the clinicians can analyses the reformatted CT study directly on their computer and simulate implant placement. The interactivity produced treatment plans can be stored or printed for future reference.[43,52]

ADVANTAGES OF SIMPLANTS

1. Stimulation of implant placement: with the help of SimPlant software program the implant can be dragged into position on a potential implant receptor site. The implant is displayed immediately in all three planes. On the cross

sectional views implants is placed in centers in the proposed site and its image declines on neighboring cross sectional views.[5]

2. Analysis of bone volume: SimPlant helps in measuring the thickness and the height of the bone up to the first anatomic obstacle. E.g. sinus, nasal fossa, mandibular canal and mental foramen. It helps to telling that

   a. atleast 2mm of safe zone must be left between the implant and anatomic structure.
   b. atleast 2mm must be left between two abutments (implants).
   c. implant angulation must exceed 30 degree to the prosthetic axis[25].

3. Analysis of bone quality: it determines the proper oesteoindication between the implant and the bone. It helps to determine the height of the selected implant and the nature of the bone. So ultimately it helps the post operative verification and ultimately leading to clinical success of the surgical procedure.[42]

4. Image Manipulation: by the variation of windows and gray scale SimPlants facilitate identification of anatomical features that are difficult to depict with a bone window. E.g. visualization of mandibular canal can be enhanced by highlighting it in colour of panaromic view.

5. Simulation of sinus grafts: SimPlants helps in telling that grafts contours must be well delimited and regular. The graft bone must be sufficient for the post operative success. The graft should be intimately related to the receptor bone and should have got no reaction with implant material.[57]

6. Analysis of implant biomechanics

This program is easy to use in dental office by the implant clinicians and requires only a personal computer working within windows. It is the most complete and accurate tool for pre operative workup of implant candidates.

Ikumi N., Tsutsumi S. et al ,(2003) conducted a study to predict the initial stability (bone quality) during implant placement by pre-surgical CT scan examination and determining whether it can be quantified. The study sample consisted of 13 subjects with 56 implants. Sites for implant placement were determined based on CT data using implant planning software. The average CT values of the bone surrounding the simulated implants were calculated by the software. Using a stereolithographic drill guide, implants were placed at the locations indicated by the protocol. The cutting torque values required for self tapping were measured during implant placement. The resulting CT values and cutting torque values were analyzed statistically for correlation. Results showed that the correlation was considered significant at a level of 0.01 or less and the correlation coefficient was 0.77. So it was concluded that strong correlation between CT values and cutting torque values in the clinical cases evaluated. These results indicate that it may be possible to predict and quantify initial implant stability and bone quality from pre-surgical CT diagnosis and implant simulation. Pre-surgical CT examination may be an effective technique for predicting initial stability of the implant and bone quality.

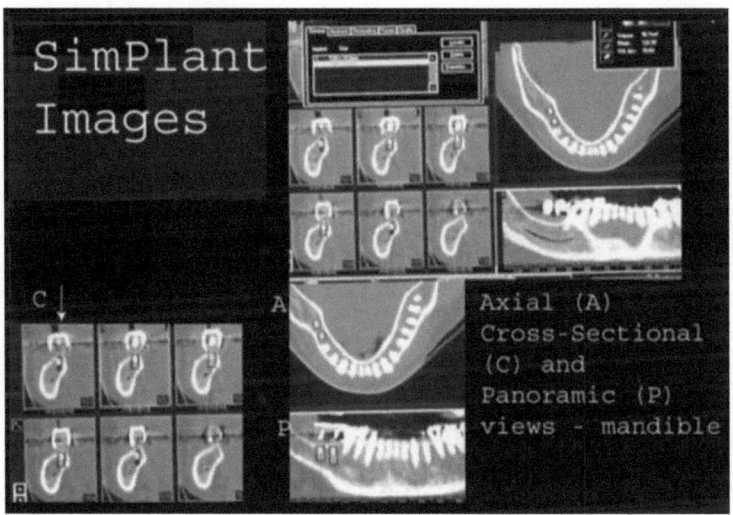

SCAN-ORA

Scan-ora is an example of a new generation of sophisticated tomographic devices most similar to conventional DPT machines, but with facilities to generate high quality sectional images. In contrast to CT scanning where the sectional images are software generated, the Scan-Ora produce a tomographic image directly onto film. It uses complex broad beam spiral tomography and is able to scan in multiple planes. The scans are computer controlled with automatic execution but still rely heavily on good patient positioning and experience in using the machine. The patient's head is carefully aligned within the device and this position recorded with skin markers and light beams. A DPT image is produced from which the sites which require sectional tomographic data are determined. The patient is repositioned in exactly the same alignment and the appropriate tomographic programme selected for the chosen region of the jaw. The Scan-Ora magnification is 1.3 or 1.7 for routine DPTs but is 1.7 for all sectional images. Tomographic sections are normally 2 mm or 4 mm in thickness. As with all tomograms the image produced includes adjacent structures which are not within the focal trough which therefore appear blurred and out of focus. Because the scan sections are thicker and fewer the overall patient dose is much less than a CT scan. The amount of detailed information provided is considerably less than a CT scan but is usually sufficient for all but the most complex cases. In order to facilitate planning using images at different magnifications, transparent overlays depicting implants of various lengths and diameters at the corresponding magnifications can be superimposed directly on the radiograph. These provide a simple method of assessing implant sites and implant placement at different angulations[54].

CONE BEAM COMPUTED TOMOGRAPHY (CBCT)

CBCT is capable of providing sub-millimeter resolution in images of high diagnostic quality, with short scanning times (10–70 seconds) and radiation dosages reportedly up to 15 times lower than those of conventional CT scans. Increasing availability of this technology provides the dental clinician with an imaging modality capable of providing a 3-dimensional representation of the maxillofacial skeleton with minimal distortion. CBCT allows the creation in "real time" of images not only in the axial plane but also 2-dimensional (2D) images in the coronal, sagittal and even oblique or curved image planes — a process referred to as multiplanar reformation (MPR). In addition, CBCT data are amenable to reformation in a volume, rather than a slice, providing 3-dimensional (3D) information. CBCT scanners are based on volumetric tomography, using a 2D extended digital array providing an area detector. This is combined with a 3D x-ray beam[54].

The cone-beam technique involves a single 360° scan in which the x-ray source and a reciprocating area detector synchronously move around the patient's head, which is stabilized with a head holder. At certain degree intervals, single projection images, known as **"basis"** images, are acquired. These are similar to lateral cephalometric radiographic images, each slightly offset from one another. This series of basis projection images is referred to as the projection data.[20,43]

Software programs incorporating sophisticated algorithms including back-filtered projection are applied to these image data to generate a 3D volumetric data set, which can be used to provide primary reconstruction images in 3 orthogonal planes (axial, sagittal and coronal). Although the CBCT principle has been in use for almost 2 decades, only recently with the development of inexpensive x-ray tubes, high-quality detector systems and powerful personal computers — have affordable systems become commercially available. Beginning with the NewTom QR DVT 9000 (Quantitative Radiology s.r.l., Verona, Italy)4 introduced in April 2001, other systems include CB MercuRay (Hitachi Medical Corp., Kashiwa-shi, Chiba-ken, Japan), 3D Accuitomo – XYZ Slice View Tomograph (J. Morita Mfg Corp., Kyoto, Japan) and i-CAT (Xoran Technologies, Ann Arbor, Mich., and Imaging Sciences International, Hatfield, PA).[49,61]

These units can be categorized according to their x-ray detection system. Most CBCT units for maxillofacial applications use an image intensifier tube (IIT)–charge coupled device. Recently a system employing a flat panel imager (FPI) was released (i-CAT).[7,8] The FPI consists of a cesium iodide scintillator applied to a thin film transistor made of amorphous silicon. Images produced with an IIT generally result in more noise than images from an FPI and also need to be preprocessed to reduce geometric distortions inherent in the detector configuration.

The various techniques used for imaging in CBCT are:[52,53]

1) **Oblique planar reformation:** This technique creates non axial 2D images by transecting a set or "stack" of axial images. This mode is particularly useful for evaluating specific structures (e.g., TMJ, impacted third molars) as certain features may not be readily apparent on perpendicular MPR.

2) **Curved planar reformation:** This is a type of MPR accomplished by aligning the long axis of the imaging plane with a specific anatomic structure. This mode is useful in displaying the dental arch, providing familiar panorama like thin-slice images .Images are undistorted so that measurements and angulations made from them have minimal error.

3) **Serial transplanar reformation:** This technique produces a series of stacked sequential cross-sectional images orthogonal to the oblique or curved planar reformation. Images are usually thin slices (e.g., 1 mm thick) of known separation (e.g., 1 mm apart). Resultant images are useful in the assessment of specific morphologic features such as alveolar bone height and width for implant site assessment, the inferior alveolar canal in relation to impacted mandibular molars, condylar surface and shape in the symptomatic TMJ or evaluation of pathological conditions affecting the jaws.

4) **Multiplanar volume reformations:** Any multiplanar image can be "thickened" by increasing the number of adjacent voxels included in the slice. This creates an image that represents a specific volume of the patient. The simplest technique is adding the absorption values of adjacent voxels, to produce a "ray sum" image. This mode can be used to generate simulated panoramic images by increasing the slice thickness of curved planar reformatted images along the dental arch to 25–30 mm, comparable to the in focus image layer of panoramic radiographs.

Alternatively, plain projection images such as lateral cephalometric image can be created from full thickness (130–150 mm) perpendicular MPR images. Another thickening technique is maximum intensity projection (MIP). MIP images are achieved by displaying only the highest voxel value within a particular thickness. This mode produces a "pseudo" 3D structure and is particularly useful in representing the surface morphology of the maxillofacial region. More complicated shaded surface displays and volume rendering algorithms can be applied to the entire thickness of the volumetric data set to provide 3D reconstruction and presentation of data that can be interactively enhanced.[25,73]

ADVANTAGES OF CBCT[54,57]

CBCT is well suited for imaging the craniofacial area. It provides clear images of highly contrasted structures and is extremely useful for evaluating bone.[8,9] Although limitations currently exist in the use of this technology for soft tissue imaging, efforts are being directed toward the development of techniques and software algorithms to improve signal-to-noise ratio and increase contrast. The use of CBCT technology in clinical practice provides a number of potential advantages for maxillofacial imaging compared with conventional CT:

1) **X-ray beam limitation:** Reducing the size of the irradiated area by collimation of the primary x-ray beam to the area of interest minimizes the radiation dose. Most CBCT units can be adjusted to scan small regions for specific diagnostic tasks.

2) **Image accuracy:** The volumetric data set comprises a 3D block of smaller cuboid structures, known as voxels, each representing a specific degree of x-ray absorption. The size of these voxels determines the resolution of the image. In conventional CT,

the voxels are anisotropic. All CBCT units provide voxel resolutions that are isotropic — equal in all 3 dimensions. This produces sub-millimeter resolution.

3) **Rapid scan time:** Because CBCT acquires all basis images in a single rotation, scan time rapid (10–70 seconds) and comparable with that of medical spiral MDCT systems.

4) **Dose reduction:** Published reports indicate that the effective dose of radiation (average range 36.9–50.3 microsievert [μSv])10–14 is significantly reduced by up to 98% compared with "conventional" fan-beam CT systems (average range for mandible 1,320–3,324 μSv; average range for maxilla 1,031–1,420 μSv).10,11,15–17 This reduces the effective patient dose to approximately that of a film-based periapical survey of the dentition (13–100 μSv)18–20 or 4–15 times that of a single panoramic radiograph (2.9–11 μSv).[5,20]

5) **Display modes unique to maxillofacial imaging** Reconstruction of CBCT data is performed natively by a personal computer. In addition, software can be made available to the user, not just the radiologist, either via direct purchase or innovative "per use" licence from various vendors (e.g., Imaging Sciences International). This provides the clinician with the opportunity to use chair-side image display, real-time analysis and MPR modes that are task specific.

6) **Reduced image artifact:** With manufacturers' artifact suppression algorithms and increasing number of projections, our clinical experience has shown that CBCT images can result in a low level of metal artifact, particularly in secondary reconstructions designed for viewing the teeth and jaws

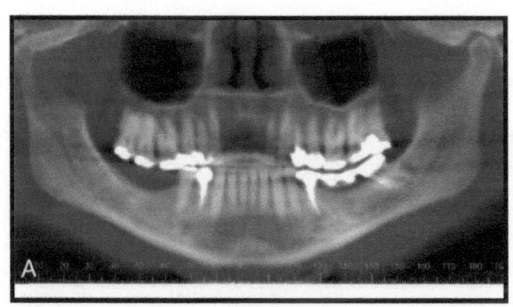

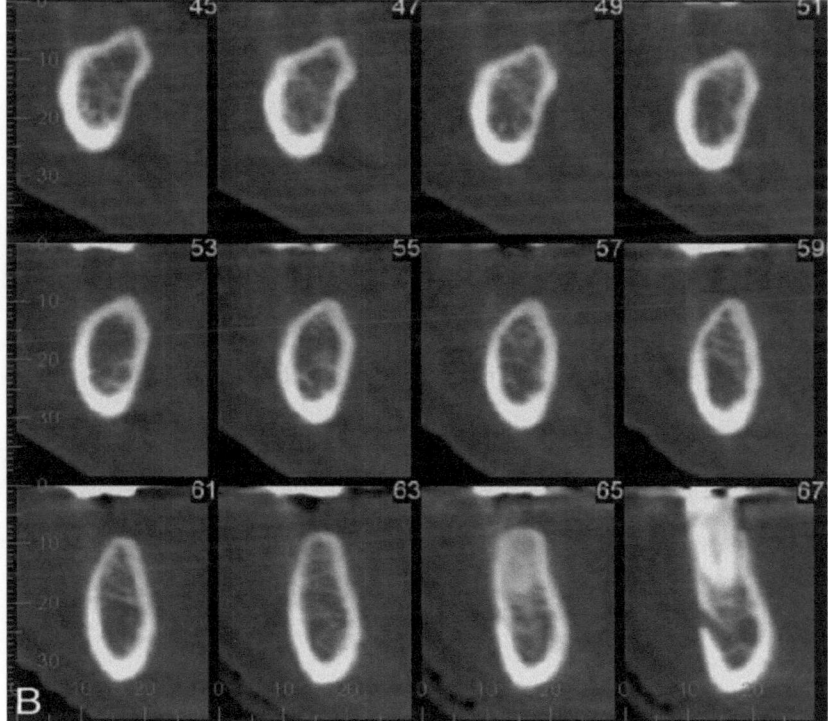

A coned-beam computerized-tomography study performed with the i-CAT 3-D imaging technology (Imaging Sciences International, Hatfield, Pa). Images are shown in 2 dimensions: (A) panoramic slice and (B) cross sections or slices. Note the mandibular canal depicted in slices 45 to 65 and the mental foramen in slice 67. These cross sections correspond to the patient's lower right edentulous region

CONCLUSION

The purpose of implant imaging is to assist the implant team in restoring the patient's occlusion and function by providing accurate and reliable diagnostic information on the patient's anatomy at the proposed implant sites.

Many radiographic projections are available for implant imaging. Intraoral, panoramic and cephalometric radiography may be used best during initial phase of patient evaluation. Once the decision for implant placement has been made, the proposed site must be further evaluated using conventional tomography or CT. MRI is not commonly used for implant imaging because bony detail cannot be readily appreciated. The cost of the procedure and radiation dose should also be weighed to the benefit of anticipated information. Clinicians should understand the indications, applications, and limitations of different imaging techniques in order to obtain maximum information while keeping radiographic risks to a minimum.[54,61]

To conclude, the imaging modalities that exist today can enhance the success and satisfaction with implant placement. Selection of projection should be made with consideration to the type and number of implants, location and surrounding anatomy. As in the case of all imaging, appropriate selection criteria must be applied individually to each patient.[16]

BIBLIOGRAPHY

1. **Abrahams JJ**. Dental CT imaging: a look at the jaw. *Radiology* 2001; 219(2): 334–45.
2. **Aguair M**. Accuracy of magnetic resonance imaging compared with computed tomography for implant planning. *Clin. Oral Impl. Res.* 2008; 19: 362–365.
3. **Akdeniz B, Oksan T, Kovanlikaya I, Genc I** . Evaluation of bone height and bone density by computed tomography and panoramic radiography for implant recipient sites. *J Oral Implantol.* 2000; 26(2): 112-8.
4. **Almog MD, LaMar J, LaMar FR, LaMar F** . Computerized tomography–based imaging and surgical guidance in oral implantology. *J Oral Implantol.* 2006; 32(1): 14-19.
5. **Almog MD**. Cone beam computerized tomography based dental imaging for implant planning and surgical guidance, part 1: single implant in the mandibular molar region. *J Oral Implantol.* 2006; 32(2): 77-82.
6. **Amet ME**. Computerized tomography with CT models for contemporary ramus frame implant planning and construction. *J Oral Implantol.*1998; 24(3): 152-60.
7. **Annibali S**. The Role of the Template in Prosthetically Guided Implantology. *J Prosthodont* .2009; 18: 177–183.
8. **Bambini F, Meme L, Procaccini M, Rossi B, Muzio LL**. Bone Scintigraphy and SPECT in the Evaluation of the Osseointegrative Response to Immediate Prosthetic Loading of Endosseous Implants: A Pilot Study. *Int J Oral Maxillofac Implants.* 2004; 19: 80–86
9. **Bhat S, Shetty S, Shenoy KK**. Imaging in Implantology. *J Indian Prosthodontic Society.* 2005; 5: 10-14.
10. **Brief J**. Accuracy of image-guided implantology. *Clin. Oral Impl. Res.* 16, 2005; 495–501.
11. **Brooks SL**. Computed tomography: *DCNA* 1993; 37: 575-90.
12. **Chau A**. Comparison between the use of magnetic resonance imaging and conebeam computed tomography for mandibular nerve identification. *Clin. Oral Impl. Res.*2011; 20: 000–001
13. **Clark DE, Danforth RA, Barnes RW, Burtch ML**. Radiation absorbed from dental implant radiography: a comparison of linear tomography, CT scan and panoramic and intra-oral techniques. *J Oral Implantol* 1990; 16(3):156–64.

14. **DelBalso AM, Greiner FG, Licata M**. Role of diagnostic imaging in the evaluation of the dental implant patient. *Radiographics* 1994; 14(4): 699–719
15. **Diniz A, Mendonca EF, Leles CR, Guilherme AS.** Changes in the pre-surgical treatment planning using conventional spiral tomography. *Clin. Oral Impl. Res.* 19, 2008; 249–253
16. **Dula K, Mini R, Stelt PF, Buser D**. The Radiographic Assessment of Implant Patients: Decision-making Criteria. *Int J Oral Maxillofac Implants.*2001; 16: 80–89.
17. **Ekestubbe A, Grondahl K, Grondahl HG**. The use of tomography for dental implant planning. *Dentomaxillofac Radiol* 1997; 26(4): 206–13.
18. **Fatemitabar AS**. Multichannel computed tomography versus cone-beam computed tomography: linear accuracy of in vitro measurements of the maxilla for implant placement. *Int J Oral Maxillofac Implants* 2010; 25: 499–505.
19. **Flyod P, Palmer P, Palmer R.** Radiographic techniques.BDJ 1999; 187(7): 123-7.
20. **Fortin T, Champleboux G**. Precision of transfer of preoperative planning for oral implants based on conebeam CT-scan images through a robotic drilling machine: *Clin Oral Implants Res* 2002; 13: 6-12.
21. **Frederiksen NL**. Diagnostic imaging in dental implantology: *Oral Surgery Oral Medicine Oral Pathology* 1995; 80: 540-54.
22. **Frederiksen NL, Benson BW, Sokolowski TW**. Effective dose and risk assessment from computed tomography of the maxillofacial complex. *Dentomaxillofac Radiol* 1995; 24(1): 55–8.
23. **Grey CF, Red path TW, Somith FW**. Low field Magnetic Resonance imaging for Implant Dentistry. *Dentomaxillofacial Radiol.* 1998; 27: 225 - 29.
24. Glossary of Prosthodontic Terms(GPT-8). *J Prosthet Dent* 2005; 94; 1-30.
25. **Harris D.E.** A.O. Guidelines for the use of Diagnostic Imaging in Implant Dentistry. *Clin. Oral Impl. Res,* 2002; 13:566–570.
26. **Hatcher CD**. Operational principles for cone-beam computed tomography. *JADA* 2010;141; 3S-6S
27. **Howerton BW and Mora MA**. Advancements in Digital Imaging: What Is New and on the Horizon? *JADA* 2008; 139; 20S-24S.

28. **Iplikcioglu H, Alca K, Cehreli MC**. The use of computerized tomography for diagnosis and treatment planning in implant dentistry. *J Oral Implantol* 2002; 38(1):29-36.
29. **Ito K, Gomi Y**. Clinical application of a new compact CT system to assess 3-D images for the preoperative treatment planning of implants in the posterior mandible: *Clin Oral Implants Res* 2001; 12: 539.
30. **Jayadevappa SB, Kodhandarama GS, SantoshV**. Imaging of dental implants *Journal of Oral Health Research*, 2010; 1(2): 50-62.
31. **Kantor ML**. Dental digital radiography. *JADA* 2005; 136: 1360-1363.
32. **Kassebaum DK, McDowell JD**. Tomography: *DCNA* 1993; 37: 567-74.
33. **Kavadella A, Karayiannis A, Karayianni KN**. Detectability of experimental peri-implant cancellous bone lesions using conventional and direct digital radiography. *Australian Dental Journal* 2006; 51(2): 180-186.
34. **Kircos LT, Misch CE**. Diagnostic Imaging and Techniques. In Misch CE editor. Contemporary Implant Dentistry, 2nd edition, St. Louis, Bosto, London, Philadelphia; 1999
35. **Kircos LT, Misch CE**. Diagnostic Imaging and Techniques.Dental Implant Prosthetics2005.
36. **Klein M, Abrams M**. Computer-guided surgery utilizing a computer milled surgical template. *Pract Proced Aesthet Dent* 2001; 13(2): 165–9.
37. **Kobayashi K et al**. Accuracy in Measurement of Distance Using Limited Cone-Beam Computerized Tomography. *Int J Oral Maxillofac Implants* 2004; 19: 228–231.
38. **Koong B**. Cone beam imaging: is this the ultimate imaging modality? *Clin. Oral Impl. Res.* 2010; 21: 1201–1208.
39. **Kraut AR and Babbush**. Radiographic evaluation of implant candidate. *In Babbush. Dental implants: art and science.35-58.*
40. **Kuhl S**. Three dimensional analysis of bone formation after maxillary sinus augmentation by means of micro-computed tomography: a pilot study. *Int J Oral Maxillofac Implants* 2010; 25: 499–505.
41. **Lindhe C, Petersson A, Rohlin M**. Assessment of the trabecular pattern before endosseous implant treatment and diagnostic outcome of Periapical radiography

in the mandible. *Oral Surg Oral Med Oral Pathol Oral Radiol Endod.* 1996; 82: 335 - 43.

42. **Li KT**. Computed Tomography in Dentistry. *Dental Bulletin2008*; 13(11); 4-8.

43. **Lal K**. Use of Stereolithographic Templates for Surgical and Prosthodontic Implant Planning and Placement. Part I. The Concept: *J Prosthodont* 2006; 15: 51-58.

44. **Mallya SM, Potluri A**. Diagnostic imaging for implants: *JIAOMR* 2004; 16: 174-80.

45. **Miles DA, Van ML**. Implant radiology: *DCNA* 1993; 37: 645-65.

46. **Mupparapu M, Singer SR**. Implant imaging for the dentist. *J Can Dent Assoc.* 2004; 7 (1): 32 – 32.

47. **Naitoh M, Katsumata A**. Measurement accuracy of reconstructed 2-D images obtained by multi-slice helical computed tomography: *Clin Oral Implants Res*2004; 15: 570.

48. **Patel N**. Integrating Three-Dimensional Digital Technologies for Comprehensive Implant Dentistry. *JADA* 2010;141; 20S-24S.

49. **Parks TE**. Digital radiographic imaging .Is the dental practice ready? *JADA* 2008;139: 477-481.

50. **Pharoah MJ**. Imaging techniques and their clinical significance. *Int J Prosthodontics*.1993; 6: 176 - 79.

51. **Potter BJ, Shrout MK**. Implant site assessment using cross-sectional tomographic image: *Oral Surgery Oral Medicine Oral Pathology* 1997;84:436-41.

52. **Rashedi B, DMD, Tyndall DA**. Tuned aperture computed tomography for cross-sectional implant site assessment in the posterior mandible: *J Prosthodont* 2003; 12: 176-82.

53. **Razavi T**. Accuracy of measuring the cortical bone thickness adjacent to dental implants using cone beam computed tomography. *Clin. Oral Impl. Res.* 21, 2010; 718–725.

54. **Reiskin AB**. Implant imaging: *DCNA* 1998; 42: 47-56.

55. **Resnik RR, Kircos LT, Misch CE**. Diagnostic Imaging and Techniques. *Contemporary Implant Dentistry.3rd edition*.pg 38-58.

56. **Rosenfeld AL, Mecall RA**. The use of interactive computed tomography to predict the esthetic and functional demands of implant-supported prostheses. *Compend Contin Educ Dent* 1996; 17(12): 1125–8.
57. **Sawyer-Glover AM, Shellock FG**. Pre-MRI procedure screening:recommendations and safety considerations for biomedical implants and devices. *J Magn Reson Imaging* 2000; 12(1): 92–106.
58. **Scarfe WC**. Clinical Applications of Cone-Beam Computed Tomography in Dental Practice. *J Can Dent Assoc* 2006; 72(1):75–80.
59. **Schropp L**. Comparison of panoramic and conventional cross-sectional tomography for preoperative selection of implant size. *Clin. Oral Impl. Res.* 22, 2011; 424–429.
60. **Schneider D**. A systematic review on the accuracy and the clinical outcome of computer guided template-based implant dentistry. *Clin. Oral Impl. Res.* 2009; 20: 73–86.
61. **Sennerby L, Wennerberg A**. A new microtomographic technique for non-invasive evaluation of the bone.structure around Implants: *Clin Oral Implants Res* 2001; 12: 91.
62. **Shetty V, Benson BW**. Orofacial implants. In: White SC, Pharoah MJ,editors. Oral radiology: principles and interpretation. St. Louis: Mosby,Inc.; 2000. p. 622–35.
63. **Siu A , Chu F , Chow T, Deng F**. Imaging modalities for preoperative assessment in dental implant therapy: An overview. *Hong Kong Dent J* 2010; 7: 23-30.
64. **Small BW**. Surgical templates for function and esthetics in dental implants. *Gen Dent* 2001; 49(1):30–2.
65. **Steenberghe A**. Localisation of the mandibular canal using conventional spiral tomography: a human cadaver study. *Clin. Oral Impl. Res.* **12**, 2001; 230–236.
66. **Stelt PF**. Better imaging. *JADA* 2008; 139; 7S-13S.
67. **Stelt PF**. Filmless imaging: The uses of digital radiography in dental practice. *JADA* 2005:136:1379-86
68. **Truhlar RS, Morris HR, Ochi S**. A review of panoramic radiography and its potential use in implant dentistry. *Implant Dent* 1993; 23: 126-32.
69. **Vandre RH, Webber RL**. Future trends in dental radiology: *Oral Surgery Oral Medicine Oral Pathology* 1995; 80: 471-8.

70. **Vasak C**. Computed tomography-based evaluation of template (NobelGuidet)-guided implant positions: a prospective radiological study. *Clin. Oral Impl. Res*.2011; 22: 1157–1163.
71. **Veigas V**. Transference of virtual planning and planning over biomedical prototypes for dental implant placement using guided surgery. *Clin. Oral Impl. Res*. 2010: 21; 290–295.
72. **Webber RL, Horton RA**. Comparison of film, direct digital and TACT images to identify the location of crestal defects around endosseous titanium implants. *Oral Surgery Oral Medicine Oral Pathology* 1996; 81: 480-90.
73. **Weinberg AL**. CT scan as a radiologic data base for optimum implant orientation. *J Prosthet Dent* 1993; 69: 381-5.
74. **Worthington P, Rubenstein J, Hatcher D**. The role of cone-beam computed tomography in the planning and placement of implants. *JADA* 2010; 141; 19S-24S.
75. **Wyatt CC, Pharoah MJ**. Imaging techniques and image interpretation for dental implant treatment. *Int J Prosthodont* 1998; 11(5): 442–52.
76. **Zabalegui J, Gil JA, Zabalegui B**. Magnetic resonance imaging. *Implant Dent* 2000; 23: 128-36.
77. **Zitzmann NU et al**. Patient assessment and diagnosis in implant treatment: *Australian Dental Journal* 2008; 53: S3–S10.